Pediatric Dramatherapy

of related interest

Medical Art Therapy with Children
Edited by Cathy Malchiodi
Foreword by Richard Lippin
ISBN 1 85302 678 6

Play Therapy
Where the Sky Meets the Underworld
Ann Cattanach
ISBN 1 85302 211 X

Essays in Drama Therapy
The Double Life
Robert J. Landy
ISBN 1 85302 322 1

Practical Approaches to Dramatherapy
The Shield of Perseus
Madeline Andersen-Warren and Roger Grainger
ISBN 1 85302 660 3

Using Interactive Imagework with Children
Walking on the Magic Mountain
Deborah Plummer
ISBN 1 85302 671 9

Symbols of the Soul
Therapy and Guidance Through Fairy Tales
Birgitte Brun, Ernst W. Pedersen and Marianne Runberg
ISBN 1 85302 107 5

Reflections on Therapeutic Storymaking
The Use of Stories in Groups
Alida Gersie
ISBN 1 85302 272 1

Pediatric Dramatherapy
They Couldn't Run, So They Learned To Fly

Carol E. Bouzoukis

Foreword by Robert J. Landy

Jessica Kingsley Publishers
London and Philadelphia

The author and the publishers gratefully acknowledge permission to reprint extracts from the following:

Adler, D. and Hull, R.F. (eds) (1967) *The Collected Works of C.G. Jung, vol. 13: Alchemical Studies.* New Jersey: Princeton University Press.

Cummings, E.E. (1959) *100 Selected Poems.* New York: Grove Press, Inc.

Thoreau, H.D. (1980) *A Week on the Concord and Merrimack Rivers: The Writings of Henry David Thoreau.* New Jersey: Princeton University Press.

Tolkien, J.R.R. (1982) *Fellowship of the Ring.* Boston: Houghton Mifflin, Co.

Penrose, R. (1983) *Picasso: His Life and Work.* Berkeley: University of California Press.

First published in the United Kingdom in 2001 by
Jessica Kingsley Publishers Ltd,
116 Pentonville Road, London
N1 9JB, England
and
325 Chestnut Street,
Philadelphia PA 19106, USA.

www.jkp.com

Library of Congress Cataloging in Publication Data
A CIP catalog record for this book is available from the Library of Congress

British Library Cataloguing in Publication Data
A CIP catalogue record for this book is available from the British Library

ISBN 1 85302 961 0

Printed and Bound in Great Britain by
Athenaeum Press, Gateshead, Tyne and Wear

To my father and mother, Dr James K.
and Ms Delores T. Bouzoukis, for inspiring me to explore
the unknown while fostering the hopes and the dreams of truth for
those who cannot...all in a place that is faraway, yet ever-present,
personal, yet universal and sometimes frightening but safe. For it is,
after all, only if you and yours believe...

Contents

Illustrations

Acknowledgments

I would first like to acknowledge the courage of the young patients, who unknowingly revealed so much of themselves in such a selfless manner. My thanks to these children for so readily illustrating the power of dramatic play. Also, my gratitude goes to the staff of the hospital/school program for their support. I would like to thank psychologist Dr Thomas Kneavel who continues to be a much-needed advocate for the ever-emerging and progressive field of dramatherapy.

My special thanks go to Dr Robert Landy, Director of the Drama-therapy Program at New York University, for his guidance over the years and for his wisdom and contribution to the field of dramatherapy. I should like to express my genuine appreciation to Dr Landy for so eloquently writing the Foreword for this, my first book. My appreciation also goes to Dr Lowell Swortzell and Dr Alistair Martin-Smith of New York University for their continuous encouragement and belief in my work.

My sincere thanks go to my illustrator, Laurence Muleh, for capturing the essence of my work through his artistry. Laurence has the ability to empathize with the children's struggles and in doing so has preserved the dramatherapy through his illustrations.

I also appreciate the effort that my local editor, Doug Gelbert, made in reviewing my ever-evolving manuscript. This book would not be possible if not for the countless hours that my typist spent – thank you, Wendy Tricarico. I would very much like to thank Stephanie Petrone for her help in typing the original manuscript, and Dr Cynthia Wiles was most helpful regarding the statistical analysis. A special thank you to Jessica Kingsley Publishers for their progressive thinking and most particularly to both Helen Parry and Emma Woolf for their support and keen insight.

Most importantly, thank you to my parents, family and friends for being there along the journey.

Foreword

For centuries philosophers and poets have served up the metaphor of the world as stage. Most likely they were catering to the tastes of grown-ups who might have been dubious of such a romanticized version of reality, having long ago exchanged the dramatic world of the imagination for that of logic and consequence. If their audience were that of children, however, their metaphor would have been most heartily applauded. Children have easy access to the imaginary realm and function very comfortably in a dramatic world, one that is celebrated regularly in children's literature by the likes of the Brothers Grimm, Hans Christian Andersen, Dr Seuss and Maurice Sendak.

As a drama educator and therapist, I think of that world as populated by heroes and villains, monsters and fairies, fools and wise folk. In fact, as I am writing this piece, my 11-year-old daughter calls me from her room to say: 'Dad, there's a monster under my bed. It has two red eyes that are glowing.' I respond by asking two questions: 'Is it a friendly monster? Does it have a name?' As I engage in my daughter's world, I leave behind for a moment my adult need to explain away the unexplainable. There is a monster under her bed and by communicating that dramatic reality, she allows me the privilege of entering her world. Little does she know that she has also entered mine, helping me write this Foreword to a book that I care very much about.

Children's drama takes place on many stages in the world – under beds, in playgrounds and dollhouses, in attics and basements. It also takes place in the mind, as children sift through a day's experience and cast their parents and siblings in the roles of friends and foes. A most special setting for children's dramas, especially young children, is the body. The world as body (*theatricum corpi*) in many ways precedes the adult notion of the world as stage (*theatricum mundi*). In terms of biological reality, the child experiences the most dramatic conflicts upon this stage. Most children can cite truly exciting struggles with tight shoes and growing feet, irascible loose teeth, out of control voices and all kinds of excitement around the taking in and elimination of food. Most all children feel from time to time like dwarves in a land of giants and tricksters, in a land of despots.

There is good reason why so many of the protagonists and antagonists of children's fairy tales, fables and legends are those whose bodies transform, deform and reform. The reason is because these characters mirror the reality of children who throughout their first 15 years of life experience such dramatic biological changes.

For some children, however, the normal developmental pattern is disrupted. Pulled into the adult world of medicine, they are encouraged to abandon their fantasies and implement the rational strategies given by their doctors, therapists and parents. The lucky ones will meet up with helpers who will recognize that the child dependent upon machines and pills also has the need to retain a connection to the inner life of images. For it is on that stage, located somewhere between the mind and the body, where miraculous, mysterious and at times healing dramas can be enacted.

The children who appear in this book were all very lucky to have found Carol Bouzoukis, a dramatherapist specializing in pediatrics. Dr Bouzoukis is a builder of bridges whose materials are stories created for and by children that span the shores of medicine and imagination. The pill that Dr Bouzoukis offers is a role, a character in a story that once ingested helps the child discover a way to feel more complete and in control.

In this book, we are introduced to several unforgettable children, like 6-year-old Caitlin, so frail that she could hardly walk or talk, dependent upon sophisticated medical treatment around the clock. Through creating the role of a soaring bird in her dramatherapy sessions, she is able for a time to transcend her physical limitations and fly uninhibitedly through an endless expanse of sky.

Because 7-year-old Tasha suffers from a severe form of diabetes, she can neither participate in active play nor enjoy the kinds of treats that her peers take for granted. In creating the role of the angel wolf, she is able to harness the power of her imagination and take more control of her fears of dying.

Brandon at 11 suffers from a chronic and life-threatening form of asthma. In working with characters from the stories 'The Three Little Pigs' and 'The Gingerbread Man,' Brandon discovers ways to breathe life into his wounded body and claim his full sense of competence.

The healing potential of pediatric dramatherapy lies in trusting that children, however ill, able-bodied or disabled, have the capacity to enter a place where they can locate the qualities necessary to survive. The place is the imagination and the qualities are various – courage, mobility, control, humor, playfulness, cunning, breath and strength and the ability to soar. It is not hard for children to find that place. But it is hard for many grown-ups, even those who are in the roles of helping children in need. When the doctors and therapists and parents minimize or forget about the healing power of the imagination, they compromise their ability to help the children they need to reach.

Dr Bouzoukis does not admonish all of us who work with children in need to abandon our conventional forms of healing through medicines and words. Rather, she reminds us to let go of the thought that these technologies are sufficient in themselves and to trust that children will go where they need to go in their search for mastery. Our job, suggests Dr Bouzoukis, is to guide them there. In providing stories and encouraging dramatic enactments, Dr Bouzoukis is a powerful and gentle guide.

When my daughter was very young, she became enchanted with the story of Cinderella. Throughout her childhood, when she was most disturbed by the limitations of her body and dark figures of her mind, she would ask for a tailor-made Cinderella story that somehow represented her struggles. The stories were good medicine for her, but now that she is growing out of childhood, their shelf life has expired. She wants more scientific explanations of how and why things work. And yet there is still that monster under the bed to reckon with.

Dr Bouzoukis reminds all professional therapists and grown-ups to heed that monster. It is real and it is scary. It lives in the minds and bodies of all children and all adults who once were children. It needs recognition, engagement, dialogue. It needs to be allowed out from

under the bed or it will lurk and fester and cause great pain. Heeding the
monster offers a way into the minds of children. Heeding the monster
with the glowing red eyes offers a way out into the physical world,
where children can summon up their courage to confront the monsters
of illness and fear. Not all children can run. But all children can fly.

Robert J. Landy

CHAPTER I

An Introduction

I had the opportunity to work at a New York City area hospital with chronically and terminally ill children during a dramatherapy internship several years ago. Although at that time I had previously worked with abused children in the mental health field, this was my first encounter with pediatric patients. The unit director took me aside on my first day and said, 'You do realize that some of these children could die?' For a fleeting moment, I wondered whether I was indeed strong enough to work with dying children. However, when I met and began working with a young cancer patient, I realized that her spirit and passion for life were nothing less than inspirational. Most of these children were so severely ill, yet they had a leashed energy that needed to be freed.

Some of the children were dying as the illness attacked them physically, but they needed a way to fight back both physically and emotionally. The children's emotions needed to be expressed. In fact, the phrase 'terminally ill' is no longer used with children because it connotes a finality, negating a hope that lives. The positive impact of this earlier experience encouraged me to work in Pediatrics years later. This more recent and challenging experience has culminated in this book. It was with the children's hope and inspiration that this book was written.

Most dramatherapy books describe techniques and methods that are designed specifically for work with adult clients. Many existing texts focus on group work in the mental health field. This book concentrates on individual dramatherapy with children in a medical setting, hence charting previously unexplored territory. Pediatric dramatherapy is a specialized and newly emerging field.

This book examines the significance of chronically ill children's role-playing by relating their fictional journeys to their own personal ones. The pediatric dramatherapy cases explored within this book are based on individual sessions. One-on-one work with this chronic population enables the therapist to focus solely on the individual's conflicts reflected through the story. Although puppets, masks, make-up and costume accessories are made available to every individual patient, it is the story that carries the child on his or her journey to self-discovery. In fact, the work described in this book is pertinent to the new and emerging field of Arts Medicine.

As a dramatherapist, I offer children a creative and natural form of self-exploration and expression through which they can examine their issues. This is done without having to process their traumas through more adult means such as direct verbalizations. Dramatherapy works in part through the unconscious, where the darkness lies. The symbolism of the stories, and more particularly that of the selected fairy tales, acts as a vehicle to transform the existing shadows into light.

This book shares my approach that has been evolving ever since I became a Nationally Registered Dramatherapist in 1987. It is an attempt to uncover the core of how dramatherapy heals the mind, body and spirit. This approach combines the use of the story drama method with the ability to interpret the connection between the fiction and the child's reality. The story drama method allows the therapist to enact a selected story almost as an informal performance for the patient. Then the child's selection of assorted people, animals or objects to become themselves establishes the groundwork where the healing begins. It is the search for meaning and the discoveries made that justify the power of dramatherapy.

This approach is strengthened by Landy's role method (1993) which provides a guideline for treatment (see Chapter 3) and helps define, through a detailed taxonomy, the very roles that are played. The use of Landy's taxonomy of roles provides pertinent information regarding the very substance and function of each role dramatized by the patients. This information acts as a catalyst for further interpretation and meaning behind the role selections.

The first case explores the world of a 6-year-old girl in need of a heart and lung transplant. Caitlin was born prematurely, weighing less than 2 pounds. When she began the dramatherapy, she was on a drug treatment program that appeared to be working, yet she needed 24-hour oxygen each day. Caitlin first presented as minimally verbal, if not inaudible. Yet she showed a marked progression due to the dramatherapy intervention. The subtitle of this book, *They Couldn't Run, So They Learned To Fly*, is particularly reflective of the first case, though not exclusively. Caitlin literally created the role of the bird where no bird existed. In the role of the bird, Caitlin flew in and out of her stories. Her need to fly was precipitated by the restrictive 24-hour oxygen tank that she constantly wheeled around on a metal frame. It was much taller than she was. Her apparent need to fly free was clear. The significance of the role of the bird and its implications for healing are further examined within this case study. This case is particularly meaningful because of the courage exhibited by such a fragile child.

Tasha is a 7-year-old child with insulin dependent diabetes. Her stories represent a silent struggle with oral restrictions due to her chronic illness. Her strict diet allowed no candy or sugars and few carbohydrates. Due to her dangerously low sugar levels she often had to sit still while the other children played. Tasha's inner frustrations were manifested symbolically within each of the tales. Her need to devour an entire gingerbread house was limitless. It much surpassed a typical child's temptation. Yet through the drama she could experience this otherwise forbidden restriction.

Because of the life-threatening nature of Tasha's illness, her original story entitled 'The Angel Wolf' gave this young girl the opportunity to explore her own mortality. How else could a 7-year-old child deal with such seemingly adult issues? Tasha was unresponsive to conventional forms of therapy, as was true of most of the participants. She was initially shy, introverted and minimally verbal. More traditional types of therapy had failed, as was indicated by the staff members themselves.

The third case concerns Brandon. He exuded mere energy through his dramatizations, which is indicative of the very live nature of this art form. His motivation to engage in acting was captured in this case study, yet reminds us of how difficult it is not only to prove the power of drama, but to capture it through words. Brandon's work was not only impressive on an artistic level, but is also an example of how the emotional and physical pain of a chronic illness can be explored symbolically through dramatherapy. Brandon has severe asthma and has been hospitalized repeatedly. He has major asthma attacks weekly, any one of which could result in death. Consequently, Brandon's physical restrictions are the cause of much anguish and frustration.

As Brandon's stories unfolded, a correlation developed between his actual respiratory problems and the physical exertion of selected characters. For example, he focuses on the huffing and puffing of the wolf and accentuates the frantic running of the gingerbread man. These are fictional forms of physical action and over-exertion. They are representative of Brandon's own severe physical restrictions in his day-to-day life. This 11-year-old boy's ability to improvise dialogue while developing solid characterizations is also reflective of the healing power of transformation. These children are able to escape their pain, if only temporarily, by becoming characters that fight unforeseen obstacles and win.

Each individual case begins with background information about the patient followed by an in-depth description and analysis. The cases themselves read almost as if they are plays. The dialogue, characters, plot twists and denouements are all an integral part of the stories as they are brought to life. This makes the cases more accessible to the reader because they often flow like a theatre script – yet, a non-fictitious script. Each case analysis is followed by a discussion and a six-month follow-up. The statistical results are presented in Appendix A. An unedited transcript of a selected session concludes every individual case. Cases 4 and 5 are summarized in Chapter 4 for review.

Dramatherapy works because it goes beyond words. As a creative form of psychotherapy, its strength lies in the power of the art form. The energy manifested by creating dramatizations in a private setting is a catalyst for self-expression. A patient's unresolved issues emerge spontaneously, often generated unconsciously through improvisational role-playing. A young patient typically either does not know the words to describe his or her plight, or selectively discloses inner feelings according to defense mechanisms. The patient may choose not to talk about his or her condition. Yet, when they're engaged in dramatic role-playing, they unknowingly explore their issues while having fun. It is the therapist's role to uncover the meaning behind the child's storymaking.

Healing must involve the treatment of the mind, body and spirit of each individual. When a child is born with a chronic illness, or develops a severe medical condition at an early age, as with the children in this book, stress is an underlying factor. In some instances, stress may be a factor relating to the cause of the illness. In other cases, the condition may precipitate stress. Often, it is both. This book is based on a study designed not only to treat children through a dramatherapy intervention, but specifically to determine the effectiveness of this modality in reducing stress.

When children assume selected roles, there is a significance to their choosing. Whether a child selects a hero (protagonist) or a beast (antagonist) to portray, it is the story that guides the characters through these inherently stressful journeys. As the child faces the stress within these dramatizations, his or her own stress may be affected. The stress level of these chronically ill children was reduced through the dramatherapy treatment, and in some cases provided a positive change in their medical condition. This book will consider these factors as the significance of this form of treatment is examined.

The challenge to the dramatherapist is to go where the child is emotionally, developmentally, and cognitively. One must always create a non-judgmental, non-threatening and private space, where a child feels free to express and be who he or she is. Always allow the child to lead you to where he or she needs to go within the drama. This includes story selection, role selection, plot development and conflict resolution. The therapist allows the child to communicate naturally through dramatic role-playing. Then the therapist analyzes, interprets and evaluates while searching for patterns and hidden meanings. The therapist becomes a detective.

Dramatherapy enables the patient the opportunity to become someone else. In doing so, defenses diminish and true selves are unknowingly revealed. By entering into a potentially transformational reality, the fiction takes form and carries the actual fears of the patients solely to resolution. The power of pretending is at the root of how dramatherapy heals.

In conclusion, this book will illustrate how dramatherapy works. It will show the reader how this artistic form of treatment can prove to be vital in meeting a sick child's unmet needs. When more traditional forms of therapy have failed or have been grossly overlooked, dramatherapy can have a positive effect on the well-being of children. The methods and techniques used in this book are readily adaptable to work with children suffering from a physical and/or emotional trauma.

Illustrations are used to enhance further the artistic significance of dramatherapy. Each illustration was originally designed by artist Laurence Muleh to capture the symbolic and often unconscious nature of this creative modality.

CHAPTER 2

Journey Through the Literature

The children who shared their stories in this book were all chronically ill patients in an area hospital, which will remain anonymous to ensure patient confidentiality. Dramatherapy, the selected treatment modality, is potentially beneficial to all hospitalized children, yet was conducted with these chronically ill patients because of the severity of their physical illness and emotional state. Siegel, Smith and Wood (1991) state: 'A chronic medical condition in children is generally assumed to be a major life stressor' (p.472).

This book explores dramatherapy specifically with children. Many of the existing and emerging dramatherapy approaches, including projective techniques, can be used successfully by young people. Dramatherapy is rooted in play and play is a child's most natural and accessible form of communication:

> The play of children exemplifies the most pure state of dramatic activity, the unmediated projection of self outwards onto the world and the concomitant assimilation of the world within the self. The ability to dramatize, to exist simultaneously within the two realities of the imagination and the objective world, marks a significant development in the growth of human consciousness. Dramatic play, as an early form of being, provides a visible shape for unconscious processes. In healthy development, the child engages in play naturally to master reality. In abnormal growth, that natural process can serve the therapeutic goal of helping dysfunctional children express their problems safely and move towards mastery. (Landy 1994, pp.66–67)

Child psychologist Eleanor Irwin (1977, 1983, 1985) specializes in dramatherapy research with emotionally disturbed children. According to Irwin: 'Drama is a method par excellence for studying the play and fantasies of children' (1981, p.427). This book applies dramatherapy to a medical setting in order to treat chronically ill children. Conventional psychotherapeutic practices have been applied to the medical model, with literature supporting 'play' techniques with medically at-risk children.

There are three major sources of stress in chronically ill children: separation anxiety, loss of control, and fear of bodily harm or death (Golden 1983; Rae and Worchil 1989; Wojtasik and Sanborn 1991). In this study, a chronically ill child took on the role of a fairy-tale character, and further dramatized the story from his or her own perspective. The expression of the stress-related issues of separation anxiety, loss of control and fear of bodily harm or death were observed by the therapist.

There is some mention in the literature that dramatherapy practices have taken place specifically in pediatric settings:

> At St. Lukes-Roosevelt Hospital Center in New York, two drama therapists, Maria Scaros and Loretto Gallo-Lopez, have worked extensively with young chronic cancer patients, using dolls and puppets to help the children express their fear of doctors, intrusive instruments, illness and death. (Landy 1994, p.140)

However, a wealth of information regarding play therapy with hospitalized children does exist. This material, combined with research on dramatherapy in mental health settings, has been examined in the review of literature with a specific focus on the dramatic play therapy (Golden 1983; Prugh 1983; Rae and Worchil 1989; Siegel *et al.* 1991).

As a drama therapist working with select chronically ill children, a single projective technique was emphasized in order to determine its specific applicability. In *Drama Therapy: Concepts, Theories and Practices* (Landy 1994), both psychodramatic and projective techniques are described in detail. Irwin (1977) considered psychodramatic techniques too direct for use with children: 'Psychodrama with children seems to be too direct (and directive), verbal, structured, reality and action oriented to help disturbed youngsters to truly work through their multiple conflicting feelings' (p.428). This does not preclude certain psychodramatic techniques from being adapted for use with children, but projective techniques promise greater value, most specifically, storytelling of the fairy tale.

Fairy tales are the specific type of stories that were examined. Their longevity, timelessness and universality are but a small reflection of their potential significance in the day-to-day world of a child. Fairy tales have recently been acknowledged for use in psychotherapy. For some children they offer a familiarity with which to begin. In *The Uses of Enchantment: The Meaning and Importance of Fairy Tales* (1975), Bruno Bettelheim supports the healing powers of fairy tales for children with a detailed exploration of their meaning from a psychoanalytic perspective:

> Applying the psychoanalytic model of the human personality, fairy tales carry important messages to the conscious, the pre-conscious, and the unconscious mind, on whatever level each is functioning at the time. By dealing with universal human problems, particularly those which pre-occupy the child's mind, these stories speak to budding ego and encourage its development, while at the same time relieving pre-conscious and unconscious pressures. (Bettelheim 1975, p.6)

A child deals with universal problems by relating to the characters of a fairy tale. When a child listens to a fairy tale, it can be therapeutic. As a child takes on a role within the fairy tale, it strengthens that therapeutic value. Sale (1978) writes, 'The crucial point about fairy tales is that they "became" children's literature but were nothing of the sort for most of their long years of existence' (p.26). Fairy tales have been used as a projective technique in therapy with adults. Robert Landy (1993), one of the pioneers of dramatherapy, has written a case study that uses *Hansel and Gretel* as a catalyst for the exploration of roles for an individual participating in group dramatherapy. In this particular case study, the client is a 30-year-old adult who chose a well-known fairy tale as her way to self-exploration through roles.

Furthermore, Birgitte Brun, a psychologist practising in Denmark, also promotes the use of fairy tales in therapy and has described in great detail their applicability in treatment: 'Fairy tales bring us into contact with pre-conscious longings and aspirations; they extend reality beyond the daily sometimes quite narrow world' (Brun, Pedersen and Runberg 1993, p.17). The authors go on to describe the actual use of fairy tales with physically ill children in a hospital.

It is, say Jacoby, Kast and Riedel (1992), the symbolism within fairy tales that offers unconscious meaning to the individual's plight: 'The psychology of the unconscious can learn a great deal from fairy tales, since they describe essential human archetypal phenomena. Jung went so far as to define fairy tales as the "anatomy of the psyche"' (pp.6–7). Both Jung and Freud championed the value of the fairy tale in providing a wealth of psychological information (Freud 1966; Jung 1964). Warner (1994) found that 'the dimension of wonder creates a huge theatre of possibility in the stories: anything can happen' (p.xvi). In order to make sense out of such a chaotic world, people turn to fairy tales for guidance.

A chronically ill child needs to know that possibilities exist in his or her own life for healing. When a child acts out a fairy tale, these possibilities can be explored. Starting at around 11 years of age children begin to understand that illness can be caused by the failure of a body part. However, children from the ages of 6 to 11 may have confused concepts of illness that include its being caused by magic or punishment (Eiser 1990). Fairy tales, because of their enchanting nature, may prove to be a revelatory venue for the child patient who is facing severe adversity.

The patients selected for this study were limited in age from 6 through 12. Dramatherapy practices have been utilized with virtually all-aged subjects, but a child's innate ability to play, and more particularly a child's need for self-expression through dramatic play, was at the core of the determination to use dramatherapy. Piaget's developmental paradigm, delineating ages four-and-a-half to seven years as the symbolic play stage of imitating and pretending, and ages 7 to 12 years as a complementary stage of the exploration of imitation, offers further guidelines for the age criteria (Piaget 1962).

In *The Dramatic Curriculum* (1980), Courtney explores the importance of drama as an integral part of a child's natural development. Between the ages of 7 and 12, the child plans his or her dramatic play through improvisation. An exploration of dramatic form transpires for children of this age group. These improvisations can be highly imaginative, as well as spontaneous and creative. This developmental stage includes the exploration of fantasy, as is the nature of fairy tales. The use of stories was limited to fairy tales which are deemed appropriate for all ages, including the elementary-age child.

The vast literature on the effects of illness and hospitalization on children makes it increasingly clear that there is considerable potential for emotional damage to children. Separation anxieties, loss of control, and misconceptions about pain and illness all combine to produce difficulties in their adjustment. Play, as the natural medium of expression and conflict resolution in children, can become the pathway to a healthy adjustment. Golden (1983) concludes: 'In spite of these research limitations, the experiences of professionals working in the field make it overwhelmingly clear that play intervention must be a regular part of the pediatric hospital program' (p.230). Dramatherapy, with its link to play and adaptability to work with children, is this therapist's choice for the psychotherapeutic treatment of chronically ill children.

This book will explore the use of fairy tales with chronically ill children, while focusing on the expression of stress-related issues. Children facing life-threatening illnesses need a way to express their fears. The struggles and obstacles faced by the sick child were reflected by selected characters' struggles within each tale. This therapist draws a parallel between the hero's struggle within the tale and the young patient's struggle with chronic illness; with special attention to related stressors. It is Zipes' (1991) opinion that the child's ability to act out or dramatize these conflicts may result in his or her own journey towards resolution:

> As long as the fairy tale continues to awaken our wonderment and enable us to project worlds counter to our present society, it will serve a meaningful social and aesthetic function, not just for compensation but for revelation: for the worlds portrayed by the best of our fairy tales are like magic spells of enchantment that actually free us. Instead of petrifying our minds, fairy tales arouse our imagination and compel us to realize how we can fight terror and cunningly insert ourselves into our daily struggles and turn the course of the world's events in our favor. (Zipes 1991)

Definitions

The following terms will be defined in order to promote a clearer understanding of this work: *drama, dramatherapy, fairy tales, chronically ill, play therapy, role, archetype* and *journey.*

Drama is the artistic modality upon which this study is based. Ritualistic drama originated when primitive man as the hunter enacted his hunt for the people of the village. According to Courtney (1989):

> The performer half-danced and half-acted in mimesis (the simple imitation of real action) and he dressed in masks and skins, mainly of the animals concerned in the hunt. By acting a hunt, and his success in it, he tried to make it come true. (Courtney 1989, p.159)

Today, drama in education is an interactive and experiential form of role-playing that is particularly well suited for children as it relates to play. The elements of drama include imitation, imagination, role-playing and interpretation (Landy 1982). Drama with children does not suggest a performance. This would become theatre. The dramatizations of this text are all enacted within the privacy of the therapy sessions and include no formal audience. According to Courtney (1980), drama is defined as:

> the human process whereby imaginative thought becomes action, drama is based on internal empathy and identification, and leads to external impersonation (both overt and covert). It is this act of impersonation that creates meaning through interaction with the external world, specifically other people. In education, such spontaneous dramatic action takes the forms of children's play, improvisation, and role-play. (Courtney 1980, p.vii)

The use of drama in this study is as a form of treatment.

Dramatherapy, a relatively recent field, was first defined by the British Association for Dramatherapists as follows:

> Dramatherapy is a means of helping to understand and alleviate social and psychological problems, mental illness and handicap; and of facilitating symbolic expression, through which man may get in touch through creative structures involving vocal and physical communication. (British Association for Dramatherapists in Landy 1994, p.58)

A more recent definition by dramatherapist Renee Emunah states:

> Dramatherapy is an active and creative form of psychotherapy that engages the person's strengths and potentialities, accesses and embraces the person's buried woundedness, and enables the practice and rehearsal of new life stances. (Emunah 1994, p.31)

Both definitions are significant because of their symbolic expression in combination with an understanding of the patient's strengths and potentialities.

A *fairy tale*, as defined by American folklorist S. Thompson, is:

> a tale of some length involving a succession of motifs or episodes. It moves in an unreal world without definite locality and definite characters, and is filled with the marvelous. In this never-never land, humble heroes kill adversaries, succeed to kingdoms and marry princesses. The fairy tale is a poetical vision of the human being and its relation to the world. For centuries this vision has given strength and confidence to the listeners, because they have felt the inner truth from it. (Brun *et al.* 1993, p.18)

The selected fairy tales for this study do not include princess themes. They do, however, include heroes fighting adversaries along a difficult journey. The fairy tale takes place in a world filled with marvel.

The children of this study are all considered to be *chronically ill*. The term 'terminally ill' is no longer used in referring to patients because of its negative connotations. Chronic illness is defined as follows:

> A disorder with a protracted course which can be fatal or associated with a relatively normal life span despite impaired physical and mental functioning. Such a disease frequently shows a period of acute exacerbations requiring intensive medical attentions. Chronic medical conditions of childhood are quite diverse and include many disease categories such as juvenile rheumatoid arthritis, diabetes, asthma, phenylketonuria, sickle cell disease, leukemia, cystic fibrosis, congenital heart disease, hemophilia and chronic kidney disease. (Siegel 1993, p.472)

All of the subjects in this study had life-threatening illnesses that were referred to as being chronic.

Play therapy, which is closely related to dramatherapy with children, was defined by the pioneer of non-directive play therapy, Virginia Axline:

> Play therapy is based upon the fact that play is the child's natural medium of self-expression. It is an opportunity which is given to the child to play out his feelings and problems just as, in certain types of adult therapy, an individual 'talks out' his difficulties. Play therapy may be directive in form – that is, the therapist may assume responsibility for guidance and interpretation, or it may be non-directive: the therapist may leave responsibility and direction to the child. (Axline 1947, p.9)

This therapist combines both non-directive and directive approaches, by directing or guiding mostly within the role.

More recently Ann Cattanach (1992a, p.69) defines the three stages of the play therapy process:

- the establishment of a relationship between the child and the therapist
- the exploration of toys, objects and dramatic play
- the development of self-esteem and a (positive) identity.

These three stages were an integrated part of this work and are described in each case.

The *role*, which is the vehicle of dramatic expression, is not only an integral part of the drama, but essential for the role method (Landy 1993) which is the selected method for this study. Psychodramatist J.L. Moreno defined role as follows:

> Role can be defined as the actual and tangible forms which the self takes. We thus define role as the functioning form the individual assumes in the specific moment he reacts to a specific situation in which other persons or objects are involved. The symbolic representation of this functioning form, perceived by the individual and other, is called role. (Moreno, in Fox 1987, p.62)

The significance of the role is explored in detail within each case and within the method section.

Archetype is another central concept to understand. According to Brun *et al.* (1993):

> Archetype – comes from the Greek *archetypon* meaning 'original.' Archetypes characterize ways of experiencing, while the instincts typify ways of acting. The archetypes form the basis of our guiding ideas... The archetypes create the possibilities of developing the archetypal images so essential in fairy tales. (Brun *et al.* 1993, p.5)

Archetypes have been described by Carl Jung as 'the unconscious images of the instincts themselves...they are patterns of instinctual behavior' (1964, p.66). Cultural mythologist Joseph Campbell states: 'Playful and unpretentious as the archetypes of fairy tale may appear to be, they are the heroes and villains who have built the world for us' (1958, p.36). As the spontaneous, unconscious and instinctual nature of the dramatherapy in this book, archetypal images will be considered.

Chetwynd (1982) describes the critical concept of *journey* as being:

> the course or direction of life as a whole. A perfectly ordinary trek can take on symbolic dimensions of value and meaning in reference to life in general. The encounters, the turning points, the crossings, the impassable barriers, reaching the destination, may all be as significant when referred to life in general, as the mythical voyages with their monstrous encounters. (Chetwynd 1982, p.228)

Dramatherapy transported the children on expeditions of self-discovery and these journeys are shared with the reader through the detailed description of each case.

The most pertinent related literature includes educational drama, dramatherapy, fairy tales and play therapy.

Educational drama

Educational drama is directly related to dramatherapy as a separate, yet influential, field. Educational drama was explored as an influential form of related literature, particularly due to its applicability to children. There are several theorists to consider, including some of the British pioneers of educational drama: Peter Slade, Brian Way, Dorothy Heathcote and Gavin Bolton. In this section, the principles of dramatic play, including the healing power of play, will be examined since play is one of the key elements that connects the fields of educational drama and dramatherapy.

Peter Slade set the stage for educational drama with his focus on play as the root of child drama. Slade (1954) defined two forms of play, personal and projected play. But more importantly, Slade tapped child drama as a form of therapy and a method of prevention. Slade recognized the significance of dramatic play as a means of developing a sense of self. He was one of the first educational drama specialists to consider the therapeutic implications of dramatic play as they relate to child drama (1954, 1995). Since dramatic play as a means of healing is at the root of dramatherapy with children, Slade's theories are therefore pertinent to this study.

Brian Way is most recognized for his contribution to the field of educational drama through his book, *Development Through Drama* (1967). Rooted in the creative process of dramatization, Way shows educational drama to be a form of personal growth and development. Not only does Way describe the applicability and value of improvisational drama, but also goes on to suggest the use of drama for personal growth:

> Throughout this book, the consistent intention of all suggestions for practical drama work has been that of helping the natural, organic development of each individual, exploring, discovering, and mastering his own resources, and attaining a sensitive, confident relationship with his environment. (Way 1967, p.268)

One's psychological wellness can be explored and shaped through the creative participation in process-oriented drama. Way's awareness of the value of drama with children as a means to personal growth, in combination with his understanding of the power of improvisation, is central to this study. All of the dramatherapy sessions involve improvisational acting, with the goal of personal growth through positive change.

The basis of this theory is further supported and advocated by both Gavin Bolton and Dorothy Heathcote, renowned educational drama specialists best known for their powerful methods of learning through doing – in this case, doing drama. Her work as a practitioner is group oriented and experiential in nature. Way's practice is rooted in the improvisational process, as is Heathcote's. However, Heathcote elevates the process with her use of role. Heathcote's use of role differs from Slade's and Way's because she teaches and guides through taking on an actual role in order to manipulate the learning process within the dramatization. Slade and Way were not directly interactive from within a role. However, the drama therapist takes on certain roles and can promote a therapeutic exchange within the role, as opposed to Heathcote's teaching in role (Heathcote and Bolton 1995).

The work of the teacher, says Wagner (1976), is carefully and expeditiously done through the dramatic roles that she enacts within the participating drama group: 'She is wholly there at every moment; her expertise is at the service of the class, but she shows it in her questioning, not in her telling' (p.97). Heathcote recognizes the universal tool of drama as a learning medium, including those with special needs.

Heathcote is unique among drama education practitioners for her work with special needs populations. She has conducted dramatizations with mentally disabled adolescents, psychotic adults, severely brain-damaged children and the visually impaired. Heathcote uses the same drama techniques with special populations that she uses with any other students. She discovers what is of interest to the group and proceeds from where she finds them. Although her goal is educational, it has social ramifications. Heathcote's technique and awareness of drama with special populations influences dramatherapy practices (Wagner 1976).

Gavin Bolton, an educational drama specialist, also believes in the process of experiencing through drama. Like Heathcote, he advocates participatory group drama with special attention to the actual roles taken on by the leader. Bolton endorses similar techniques and philosophies, viewing drama as a way of learning about life. Again there is an emphasis on the universal, communal qualities of drama, as well as a recognition of the magic that occurs when creating something that is not really happening. Bolton's *Drama as Education* (1984) and *Acting in Classroom Drama: A Critical Analysis* (1998) are both relevant sources to this study. In addition, Jonathan Neelands' *Making Sense of Drama* (1984) offers insight regarding the treatment and actual assessment of children participating in drama. *Stories in the Classroom: Storytelling, Reading Aloud, and Role-Playing with Children* (Barton and Booth 1990) is another relevant source because of its in-depth exploration of the use of stories in drama.

Nancy King's *Storymaking and Drama* (1993) is another source that supports the use of story in its ability to encourage individuals to think deeply about their own lives. Although this text is designed for secondary levels, the concepts are applicable to any age group. King uses poetry, short stories and plays as a catalyst for self-exploration and development. Special consideration is made for reflection upon the creative process within participatory group work. King's work relates to this study because of the significance of the story as the root for all drama.

Dramatherapy

Dramatherapy and the techniques, approaches and theories that are most applicable to the treatment of children are relevant. Ann Cattanach is a drama therapist and play therapist who recognizes the psychological relevance of playfulness. Her books, *Play Therapy with Abused Children* (1992a), *Drama for People with Special Needs* (1992b) and *Children's Stories in Play Therapy* (1997) advocate the healing nature of drama with a variety of populations. More specifically, Cattanach discusses the play/dramatherapy process for abused children in great detail. The actual case study descriptions offer a concrete understanding of the therapeutic process. 'The fear seems to lessen after many repeated enactments of the stories and rituals developed in play when the power of the monster vanquished' (1992a, p.79). The same holds true within the fairy tales of this study, whereas the assorted beasts are repeatedly enacted in order to lessen the fear that they provoke.

Robert Landy's pioneering work as a drama therapist and theorist is pertinent to this study. Landy's wide contribution to the field was first considered regarding the fundamentals. In *Drama Therapy: Concepts, Theories and Practices* (1994, first published 1986), Landy explored the interdisciplinary sources of dramatherapy. They play key roles in understanding dramatherapy with its particular application to a child population. Projective techniques are also explored.

Puppets, masks, make-up, dolls and costume accessories are all described as the drama therapist's tools for creation. However, the story is the connecting factor among these methods. The story itself, says Landy (1994), is the basis for the dramatization, whether it is through the use of a mask or a hat:

> Storytelling is a familiar form to most clients – children and adults alike. As an embodiment of archetypal imagery, it becomes a bridge between the heroes and demons of mythology and literature and those lurking within the unconscious mind. (Landy 1994, p.150)

Storytelling is the selected technique for this study. Storytelling is an art form that communicates ideas and experiences, so that the listener can find inspiration towards expression. Once the story is told, it is given to the client to explore first-hand through their own role-playing. Puppets, masks and make-up are other techniques made available in this study, yet the story itself is the catalyst for exploration. According to Gersie and King (1990): 'Stories and tales are the product, the end and therefore, paradoxically, the beginning of our journey towards under-standing' (p.31).

Landy's *Persona and Performance* (1993) is a critical source for this study because of his development of the dramatherapy role method and taxonomy of roles. Landy's role system provides not only a theory but also a procedure from which to work. The role method, says Landy (1993), delineates a guideline to treatment that focuses on the role itself:

> Heroes, also known as searchers, take a journey – whether a literal journeying forth into the world, or a voyage deep within the inter-nalized role system in order to make sense of their existence. The heroic journey involves a confrontation with significant dangers and threats on both a psychological and a physical level. (Landy 1993, p.160)

The hero goes in quest of these journeys and faces the antagonists. Both the protagonists and antagonists will be explored by using Landy's taxonomy of roles. This taxonomy categorizes and describes everyday roles that are found in theatre literature. Both the role method and the taxonomy of roles are rooted in role theory, which continues to be developed by Landy as a means of discovering one's identity. These journeys are described by Joseph Campbell (1972): 'although our voyage is to be outward, it is also to be inward, to the sources of all great acts, which are not out there, but in here, in us all, where the muses dwell' (p.233). The dramatherapy journey becomes an inward one.

Sue Jennings (1986, 1987, 1990, 1993, 1998) is a prolific author and dramatherapist whose works are a cornerstone of the field. Her background in anthropology enhances her extensive experience as a clinician and educator. Most pertinent to this book is her work in drama and play therapy with children.

Storymaking in Education and Therapy (Gersie and King 1990) is a rich source pertaining to the significance of the story in therapy, whether it be myth, tale or legend. This book includes a wealth of stories from around the world and step-by-step guidelines as to their implications for group work:

> Through the process of connection with the story's content, we are able to discover the personal meaning it has for us. Our psyche is nourished by the evocation, stimulation and expression of actual inner imagery. The awareness of self is enhanced through exploring these images in drama, movement, sound, writing, talking, painting and sculpting. (Gersie and King 1990, p.24)

Gersie and King advocate the use of traditional stories in therapy.

Gersie's *Storymaking in Bereavement: Dragons Fight in the Meadow* (1991) is highly pertinent to this study in that it deals with the healing powers of the story with particular attention to the issues of love and loss. This text explores cross-cultural myths and folk tales with an understanding of the universal nature of sorrow and its reflection within the safety of symbolic expression. Gersie believes that the power of story is at the root of expressive therapy. This is further explored in Gersie's *Earth Tales* (1993).

Fairy Tales

This section will concentrate on the literature related to fairy tales and their psychological implications. In Bruno Bettelheim's *The Uses of Enchantment: The Meaning and Importance of Fairy Tales* (1975) he defends the significance of the fairy tale for a child's psychological development. The parallel between the meaning of a fairy tale and the child's need to find meaning in his or her own life is analyzed. The hopes, struggles and conflicts that the young protagonist faces are directly related to the child's own universal or personal dilemmas. Bettelheim not only justifies the identification that occurs between child and character, but writes psychoanalytic essays on several well-known fairy tales. These detailed accounts of the symbolic meaning of the tales offer insight into the use of the stories in psychotherapeutic treatment.

Jungian psychologist Birgitte Brun is co-author of *Symbols of the Soul: Therapy and Guidance Through Fairy Tales* (1993). Brun explores the power of fairy tales in therapy. The distance of a story often allows for a feeling of safety in that it can offer 'an indirect way to approach themes that are difficult to talk about' (p.20). Brun advocates the use of these stories with both children and adults who are experiencing a trauma or loss. It is the rich symbolism within a greatly imaginative vehicle, such as the fairy tale, wherein lies the answers, although often it is unconscious.

Acclaimed scholar and mythologist Joseph Campbell explores the significance of the myth and fairy tale in our culture as it has been sustained for centuries. The fairy tale is not a simple form of entertainment designed to pass the time. One's fascination with the tales equates to the proportion of its symbolic content. The human mind finds immense pleasure from symbolization. According to *The Flight of the Wild Gander*:

> Its [the fairy tale] world of magic is symptomatic of fevers deeply burning in the psyche: permanent presences, desires, fears, ideals, potentialities that have glowed in the nerves, hemmed in the blood, baffled the senses since the beginning. (Campbell 1958, p.36)

Campbell goes on to say that the irrational and unnatural motifs of the fairy tale are from the reservoirs of man's dreams and visions.

Marie-Louise Von Franz, author of *The Interpretation of Fairy Tales* (1987), *The Feminine in Fairy Tales* (1993), and *Shadow and Evil in Fairy Tales* (1995) is also a Jungian analyst whose written works contribute to the related literature. Von Franz delves in great detail into the meanings of fairy tales as they relate to women, and to mankind. Von Franz interprets the symbolism of these tales in a clear and succinct manner. In addition to offering a synopsis of several tales, Von Franz describes a detailed analysis of each from a Jungian perspective. It is therefore the psychological perspectives of the aforementioned authors, as well as other prominent psychologists and literary scholars, that were considered as being pertinent to this study.

Animal symbolism is explored in *The Frog King: On Legends, Fables, Fairy Tales and Anecdotes of Animals* (Sax 1990), *Signifying Animals: Human Meaning in the Natural World* (Willis 1990) and *Picturing the Beast: Animals, Identity and Representation* (Baker 1993). These sources explore animals as a reflection of human identity, including man's projections of his deepest hopes and fears. *Animal-Speak: The Spiritual and Magical Powers of Creatures Great and Small* (Andrews 1993) examines the mystical and spiritual significance of animals as found in nature. This text goes beyond an appreciation for animals, as it promotes an understanding of their meaning in our lives. *Animal-Speak* contains several dictionaries of animals, including more specifically birds. The animal symbolism delineated in this book is pertinent in discerning the animals in the fairy tales.

Evil fairy tale characters are interpreted symbolically in *Witches, Ogres, and the Devil's Daughter* (Jacoby *et al.* 1992). The richness and depth of symbolism, as well as caution regarding role interpretation, are considered in the detailed account of the use of fairy tales in psychotherapy. Fairies and giants are similarly analyzed throughout the history of literature in *The Fairies in Tradition and Literature* (Briggs 1967). This source includes a comprehensive appendix that lists and defines types of fairies.

Play Therapy

Play therapy is considered, with special attention to 'dramatic' play therapy due to its applicability and relation to dramatherapy with children. In Courtney's *Play, Drama and Thought* (1989), drama and play are specifically analyzed as they relate to education. The symbolism expressed through play, as in a dream, holds the conflicts and possible solutions for the individual. There are several basic play therapy theorists who have pioneered this field, including Anna Freud, Melanie Klein and Virginia Axline. Anna Freud, like her father Sigmund, is psychoanalytic and considers play to be a way to promote the child's verbalization with eventual interpretations (Freud 1966). Freud's method is a direct approach of psychoanalysis for children. Freud tended to use play in order to develop an alliance between patient and therapist. She then proceeded to use direct verbal interactions within the therapy sessions (Schaefer and O'Connor 1983).

Klein used play as a substitute for verbalizations. She recognized play as a natural means of expression for children. Klein tended to interact within the role-playing while speculating to herself regarding interpretations until further clarifications took place (Committee on Child Psychiatry 1982).

Virginia Axline (1947) is a non-directive or client-centered play therapist. This philosophy is based on the works of Carl Rogers and his client-centered therapy for adults. The basic premise for client-centered therapy is that the individual holds the answers and that only he or she is responsible for discovering personal solutions: 'the client is the source of the living power that directs the growth within himself' (p.24).

Eleanor Irwin is a psychoanalytic child psychologist who advocates the use of drama in therapy. Irwin recognizes the power of dramatic play, wherein a child can express his or her conflicts, wishes and fears through the symbolization inherent in the dramatizations. Irwin has explored the use of puppets in therapy as a means of creating dramatized stories which, in turn, can be analyzed. The stories that possess multiple meanings are comparable to the mysteries of our dreams. Irwin (1983) found that: 'In a sense, the enacted story is similar to the manifest content of a dream; it is full of distortions and disguises meant to protect and obscure' (p.160). Special considerations must be made in conducting play therapy with a chronically ill child:

> The problems associated with chronic illness, such as asthma, diabetes, advanced kidney disease, leukemia, hemophilia, chronic cardiac problems, juvenile rheumatoid arthritis, sickle cell anemia, spina bifida, spinal cord injuries, or muscular dystrophy, to name a few, are serious and can affect all aspects of the child's personal development. (Elliott, Jay and Willis 1982, pp.33–34)

Chronic childhood disease will affect 10 to 15 per cent of children in the USA before they turn 18 (Siegel *et al.* 1991). Researchers have studied the psychological effects of a chronic illness and the consequential hospitalization on a child's psyche (Lubkin 1990; Roberts 1986).

There are several variables that will affect the psychological impact of a chronic illness, considered very stressful on a child. These include:

> the child's age at onset; the severity, duration, symptomatology and visibility of the illness; the type and extent of medical intervention; degree of family disruption and extent of financial burden, and individual child and parent characteristics that can moderate successful coping. (O'Dougherty and Brown 1990, p.326)

Children with a chronic medical condition can be adversely affected psychologically in terms of feeling anxiety, fear or anger, but the impact varies according to the individual rather than being based on diagnosis alone. Ruth Stein's *Healthcare for Children: What's Right, What's Wrong, What's Next?* (1997) is another valuable reference in offering insight into the realm of pediatrics.

Golden (1983) considers play therapy with chronically ill children essential as a natural form of psychotherapy: 'Play intervention for children in hospital settings is an unqualified necessity. The play therapist's puppets are every bit as important as the surgeon's knife' (p.213). For Willis *et al.* (1982) 'pediatric psychologists are most likely to use play therapy with medically ill children, especially in hospital settings' (p.56).

The dramatized play is at the center of this study. Dramatic play is a crucial part of play found in play therapy practice. Pediatric psychologists, child-life specialists and nurses often use stories, puppets or dolls to encourage dramatic role-playing with ill children. More specifically, there is literature describing the psychotherapeutic use of fairy tales with patients in medical settings (Bornstein 1988). Literature pertaining to play therapy with chronically ill children with special attention given to the dramatic play and implications for treatment is significant.

CHAPTER 3

Prelude to the Magic
The Method

Setting

A children's day hospital was the setting for the study. Through a cooperative effort between the hospital and the State Department of Public Instruction, this program is housed in the state's major teaching hospital. The children's day hospital is an actual school located in the hospital. It is designed to provide an education for young people who would normally be too ill to attend regular school. All school credits are transferred to the child's home school.

The children's day hospital is housed in what was once a unit in the hospital. Actual hospital rooms have been converted into classrooms. There is one room each for the lower, middle, and high school aged patients. A small activity room and shared offices are available. The common area, once a nurses' station and the foyer, is transformed into a lunch room or a group meeting space as needed. The staff have been resourceful in their use of such a relatively small space. Up to twenty-four patients can be admitted per semester.

This children's day program has the feel of both a school and a hospital. The staff are a combination of both hospital and school staff. Each child has a primary physician, nurse, social worker, teacher and various support staff. Medical needs are dealt with right at school. Treatment includes medications, dialysis, IVs, chemotherapy and physician visits.

The therapist first observed the children in their own setting at a town meeting, where she was introduced to the patients and staff. The town meeting is designed for all patients/students to attend, in order that they can process daily issues or concerns. The staff attend these meetings as well. The children of this partial hospitalization program range in age from 6 to 18 years. At this point the determination had not yet been made as to which children would be selected to participate in the study.

Selection of participants

The criteria for patient selection were diagnosis, age, availability, and supervisory and parental approval. All patients in the program were diagnosed with a chronic illness, satisfying the first criterion. The age for participation in the study had been determined to be 6 through 12 years of age, narrowing the available participants, as the majority of patients in the hospital were over 12 years of age. The director of psychology and the director of education discussed possible candidates. The therapist, in order to maintain objectivity, was not involved in the selection process. The director of psychology named 12 patients who would be potential candidates for the study.

The therapist next contacted parents, describing the study and distributing consent forms. After meeting the criteria for diagnosis and age, and obtaining supervisory and parental approval, the final hurdle was availability. Those children regularly attending the summer program became the participants for the experimental group. Children who met the criteria but had irregular attendance became the control group.

Methods of evaluation

The specific methods of evaluation include patients' medical charts, interviews of parents and selected staff observations and testing.

Medical charts

The therapist had access to all the patients' medical charts. The charts include the child's medical history, family status and progress notes. The progress notes are frequent and up-to-date reports; commentaries relate specifically to the patient's condition, both medically and behaviorally. Physicians, nurses, social workers, physical therapists and educators report a detailed account of their observations and findings regarding each patient. This much-needed information emanated from a varied perspective.

Interviews

The therapist scheduled interviews with parents or guardians and with staff members. The interviews were designed to gain information regarding the child's behavior with specific attention to any observable change in his or her overall behavior or stress level. Parents and staff observed the children outside the dramatherapy sessions, lending objectivity to the pertinent information for the study. The questions were also designed to elicit the child's overall feelings towards his or her dramatherapy experience. This was one indication as to whether or not the child had a positive or productive experience, which helped in establishing if stress could have been reduced. At the end of each dramatherapy session, a reflective process occurred with each child regarding the preceding dramatization. This verbalization process was out of role, and often yielded penetrating insight into the patient's experience. This informal form of interviewing was never pre-determined.

Interview questions for the adults were designed in order to allow for any spontaneous comments. All interviews consisted of open-ended questions regarding the child's physical and emotional state. A standardized open-ended interview presented the same questions to each individual, fostering consistency. Parents or guardians were contacted before the treatment in order that the study be described and to answer any questions. An interview with parents was scheduled at the completion of the dramatherapy sessions. The primary care nurse of each patient was interviewed after the dramatherapy sessions had been completed.

The primary care nurse is responsible for the daily care of each patient. This medical care includes disbursements of medications, invasive procedures, blood work, and routine monitoring of each child's condition. Each nurse is assigned permanently to several patients with whom he or she works closely five days a week. This regular contact breeds astute observations of behavioral changes in the patients.

The clinical social worker, involved with all subjects since they were admitted, was interviewed after the ten dramatherapy sessions had been done. She conducted weekly group sessions with all the patients of the unit including the adolescents. She specializes in bereavement and loss.

Case studies

A detailed analysis of three of the five dramatherapy cases is provided. They offer three distinct cases, based on three differing diagnoses. The stress level of each patient is the determining factor as to whether a change occurred during or after the dramatherapy sessions. Any changes in stress were noted based on several forms of evaluation. The particular story and character that the patient selected were considered as they relate to stress. The thematic content was reviewed based on the types of stress-related incidents enacted.

Each dramatherapy session was audiotaped and labeled with the patient's name and date. There were five cases consisting of ten sessions each. This produced 50 audiotapes. In addition, a detailed log was kept after each individual session. The log was a method of recording all observations, recurring themes and patterns. This was also mandatory in that the audiotapes alone were not a complete record of the actual observations required.

All information gained from the case studies was, therefore, recorded on the audiotapes and in the log. Stress symptoms, stress-related issues, and changes in stress were observed and recorded. The stressful events that the characters faced within the fairy tales were documented as they related to separation anxiety, fear of loss of control and fear of bodily harm or death. Three of the dramatherapy cases were fully detailed and analyzed, in order to reflect the actual experience. The use of commentaries provided an ongoing analysis of each case. Cases 4 and 5 were summarized.

Children's Manifest Anxiety Scale – Revised

The CMAS-R (Reynolds and Richmond 1978) is a self-reporting measure of stress and anxiety designed specifically for children, and was used as both a pre- and post-test. This standardized instrument is a 37-item scale, known as the 'What I Think and Feel' test. It was presented orally for young children, where each statement was read out loud and the child responded 'yes' or 'no.' The CMAS-R was administered individually to each child during the first session and the ninth. It was not given during the final session due to any anxiety which may have surfaced due to termination of the therapy. The control group was administered the test during the same time frame as the experimental group, but did not receive any dramatherapy treatment. Results for the experimental group were discussed as they applied to each individual case and then cumulatively with the results from the control group (see Appendix A).

Symptoms of Stress Measure

In addition to the CMAS-R, the therapist administered an observational stress measure based on the symptoms of stress as compiled by psychologist Michael Antoni (Pelletier 1993). According to Antoni, there are several categories of stress-related symptoms: cognitive, emotional, behavioral and physiological. Cognitive symptoms include poor concentration and difficult memory. Emotional symptoms include tension, irritability, restlessness, inability to relax and depression. Behavioral symptoms include avoidance of tasks, difficulty in completing work assignments and fidgeting. Physiological symptoms, more difficult to observe within a therapy session, include stiff or tense muscles, frequent urination and headaches or nausea.

This 13-item stress measure was administered by the therapist through observation. The therapist looked for any indication of the selected stress-related symptoms. The checklist was utilized after the second dramatherapy experience, and again after the final session. The children did not know this measure was used as they did not participate directly in responding to the symptoms. It is not a self-measure, but a tool for the therapist to use as a way to rate all observed symptoms of stress. The checklist rates all symptoms on a scale from a low of one to a high of five. Pre- and post-measure results are discussed as they pertained to each individual case study.

Procedure

Individual sessions were scheduled with each patient for an initial introductory meeting. Ten individual dramatherapy sessions were scheduled over a 12-week period for the five participating patients. The control group of five patients received no treatment. Each session was held in a small, private office, generally used by the psychology staff. Each child was offered the opportunity to participate in a drama program by the therapist. Drama was described to them as being when you act or pretend to be someone or something in a story. They were told that they would choose from five stories and could use anything in the drama bag to help them to act: puppets, masks, make-up, hats or costume accessories. If they indicated interest, the assent form was read to them. The Children's Informed Assent Document explains to the child what the study is about and how their participation would be viewed. After hearing what the form stated, the child was asked to sign his or her name if they wanted to have drama. All children were told that if at any point they no longer wanted to have drama, they could stop and that would be okay too.

After the assent forms were signed, the next step was to administer the CMAS-R assessment inventory. The findings were not evaluated until after the 12 weeks were completed. The dramatherapy sessions were then scheduled with the five patients over the course of 12 weeks. Each child participated in ten sessions, lasting no less than 30 minutes and no longer than 45 minutes, depending upon age and developmental level of the subject. The patients were asked to select one of the five available fairy tales.

The five classic and well-known fairy tales selected for use in this study were *Jack and the Beanstalk, Hansel and Gretel, Little Red Riding Hood* (Opie 1993), *The Three Little Pigs* and *The Gingerbread Man* (Leete-Hodge 1983). Each story involves a protagonist or hero who embarks on a journey while facing life-threatening obstacles. The researcher selected these tales specifically because of this common theme and its potential to relate to a child's own struggle in everyday life. Each child is on his or her own journey while facing life-threatening obstacles because of a chronic illness. The therapist selected these stories because they contained clear incidents of separation anxiety, loss of control, and fear of bodily harm or death. Furthermore, each fairy tale featured a straightforward plot with no more than five primary characters. The relative simplicity in structure and these stress-related conflicts were determining factors in the story selection.

During each individual dramatherapy session, five fairy tales were made available to the patient. After the child chose a story, the therapist acted out the story for the child. Then the patient selected a character he or she wanted to be and proceeded to act out the story with the help of the therapist. Therefore, during each session the child was given the opportunity to chose a story, listen to it, and then act it out. Story and character selection may have varied from session to session, or within a session. The stories, characters and drama materials were the constant variables which the patient and therapist worked within. The specific details and contents of each therapy session were explored as each case study evolved.

The Symptoms of Stress Measure was reviewed and rated for each child after the second session. This was done by the therapist and based on observations made since the first session. The child was not made aware of this rating, nor was he or she ever to be made aware of the specific purpose of the study itself. After the dramatherapy sessions had been completed with each patient, the CMAS-R and the Symptoms of Stress Measure were administered a second time as a post-test (see Appendix A).

The findings from all interviews that relate to the child's stressors were documented. Selected transcriptions of pertinent dialogue regarding the patient's level of stress were also highlighted. Each individual case was then analyzed for its content applicability. Landy's role method (1993), which provided not only a guideline for treatment but also for reflection and analysis, was considered:

1   Invoking the role.

2   Naming the role.

3   Playing out/working through the role.

4   (a) Exploring alternative qualities in sub-roles; (b) ability to invoke and understand counter-role.

5   Reflecting upon the role play.

6   Relating the fictional roles to everyday life.

7   Integrating roles to create a functional role system.

8   Social modeling.

These eight steps acted as a general outline in order that the child's own natural ability to dramatize be encouraged yet not restricted:

> The therapeutic actor, like the theatrical actor, is given permission to move in and out of two contiguous realities: that of the imagination, the source of unconscious imagery, and that of the everyday, the domain of grounded daily existence. (Landy 1993, p.46)

It is through this transformation into the fictional role that the patient is then able to embark on self-exploration. Discoveries are revealed only by stepping away from daily existence and into the security of a supposedly other someone. It is through this perceived distance that one's creative process allows for symbolic expression, which is both safe and revealing at once. Therefore, it was through the use of Landy's role method that the dramatherapy sessions were discussed. As noted, special attention was given to the stress-related incidents that had been previously established to exist within given roles.

Dramatherapy process

Each individual dramatherapy session consisted of an initial preparation period, the action phase and a processing phase as closure. Before each session was scheduled to begin, the therapist met with the patient wherever he or she happened to be on the unit, either in the classroom or involved with a project. Sometimes the patient was with a primary care nurse or physician. Generally, the patients seemed eager and willing to attend.

When the drama therapist and patient reached the office, where all dramatherapy sessions were held, the therapist/researcher sat at the desk and the patient sat on the office couch. At the beginning of each session, the drama therapist read the list of the five fairy tales and asked the child to select one. During the first therapy session for each child, the therapist asked whether or not the child was familiar with each story. This information was recorded, since lack of familiarity may have influenced story selection. After the story was selected, the therapist acted out the story by becoming the narrator and all of the characters. This story drama method was originally designed by the therapist for group work.

The therapist as performer allowed for a live enactment of the selected story, which helped to set the tone. By acting out the story, the therapist encouraged participation by initiating the art form. As the children watched the story, they were able to imagine themselves within the story. After the children observed the story dramatization they were asked to select who in the story they would like to be. Any person, animal or thing was available to them from which to pick.

After the story had been presented, and the child selected a character to become, he or she was then given the option of selecting any drama items from the drama bag. The children tended to explore through all of the items, as they were new to them. As the sessions evolved, the children knew which drama materials they were going to use. Each child eventually tended towards one or two specific projective techniques.

Once the child decided on his or her drama items, the drama therapist presented the option of acting out the story in whole or part. After the child decided which scene or scenes would be dramatized, the therapist asked if the child wanted the therapist to play any part. The child would tell the therapist who to be and this usually included the role of the narrator. The drama then began, with the child leading as much of the actual direction as possible. The therapist while in the role often said, 'What happens next?' or 'What should he/she do now?' or even 'What should they say?' This is similar to educational theater specialist Dorothy Heathcote's own method of engaging children in drama through specific questioning. 'She wants the children to discover as much as possible through the drama itself' (Wagner 1976, p.97). The therapist asked pertinent questions of the patient in order that they reveal their own conflicts. The patient needed to make his or her own discoveries. The child was to act out only one story per session, but could play as many roles as desired. Different drama accessories could also be used to differentiate various roles.

After the story came the processing stage. Often this was done as the drama materials were returned to their bag, or while make-up was being removed. Informal reflections were made by the therapist in order to give the child the opportunity to process thoughts or concerns regarding the enacted story. At the end of every session, the researcher told the patient when his or her next session was scheduled.

The role method was a basis for the dramatherapy treatment and evaluation. According to Landy's (1993) role method, there are eight steps to be considered as a guideline for treatment. Since this study was designed for young children aged 6 to 12, some of the steps were modified, as is noted.

Invoking the role

Each child was given a choice of selecting one story from the five available tales. After selecting any story for an individual session, the story was then presented by the therapist. Each story was based on an original version. Once the child watched the story be enacted, role was invoked by the selection of any character. Any person, animal or thing was made available to them. According to Landy: 'The invocation of the role, then, is a calling into being of that part of the person that will inspire a creative search for meaning' (1993, p.47). Usually, the child selected an actual role from the story. During each session, the child always selected a role before searching through the bag of drama objects. Although the objects may have influenced the child's choice, the therapist carefully selected a variety of accessories that could enhance the dramatization of any of the stories. At times, the child created an original role or chose a role from another story. Either way, a role was selected at the beginning of each action phase of the session. At other times the child selected several roles, or added on roles as the story evolved. The invoking of the role was always left entirely up to the child, without any suggestions or leading from the therapist. Thus the role must have stemmed from the child's needs. Often the process of taking on the role is an unconscious one: 'In some ways the role actually chooses the role player' (Landy 1993, p.47). Therein lies the power.

Naming the role

Most of the roles were already named, based on the classic fairy tales from which they were derived (e.g. Hansel and Gretel, The Gingerbread Man, Little Red Riding Hood, The Three Little Pigs). If a child created an original role, he or she was asked what its name was, usually within the improvised dialogue. Naming the role is important because the patient was able to achieve distance from the role by becoming someone other than themselves. Particularly with young children, it helps to work through a fictional role, in part due to the safety of expressing oneself while being someone else.

Playing out / working through the role

Every session involved the playing out and working through of the selected role(s). The action portion of the session, which was the majority of the session, involved the playing through of the role. The pattern of role selection and of acting through the role from session to session has been noted in each case. The stress-related issues that the selected roles faced within each story are at the root of the 'working through.' Separation anxiety, fear of loss of control and fear of bodily harm or death are the significant issues that were observed as the role(s) played out. The study was designed for individual dramatherapy, as opposed to group therapy. Therefore, the individual child was given the opportunity to work through each role while being at the focus of each session. They were able to act out their stress-related issues by working through a fictitious role that was all their own.

Exploring alternative qualities in sub-roles

Some patients would explore a certain role at an earlier stage of the dramatherapy sessions and then stay with that specific role for the remainder of the sessions. Since role selection was always left up to the child, they were able to remain in their preferred role due to its apparent significance or security. As is described in Case 4, Aaron selected the role of the Wolf during the first dramatherapy session. During the next two sessions, Aaron explored the role of the Witch and then the role of the Giant. Both of these roles were antagonistic. Yet Aaron returned to the role of the Wolf and remained in this role for the next six sessions.

More often than not, however, the patient was able to explore alternative qualities in sub-roles. One example of the exploration of a sub-role is found in the case of Tasha. As described in Case 2, Tasha was in the role of the Wolf from the story of *Little Red Riding Hood* during the ninth session. As the story unfolded according to the classic tale, Tasha as the Wolf proceeded to gobble up Grandmother and Little Red Riding Hood. But after the huntsman killed the Wolf, the story did not end. The role of the Wolf morphed into the role of the 'angel-wolf.' Tasha was trying to understand death through the sub-role of her 'angel-wolf.' She explored alternative qualities of the role of Wolf. Tasha's exploration of this sub-role allowed her to discover a significant issue. The patients were never directly told what role or sub-role to invoke. This was always left up to them. The therapist encouraged their exploration of self through role-playing only in that they knew they could be whoever they wanted to be. This process is discussed in greater detail within each of the cases in this book.

Ability to invoke and understand counter-role

During the progression of sessions within each case, the researcher was observing the specific selection of role(s) made by each patient. In addition to noting the role of choice, the counter-role representing the other side of the patient's selected part was considered. An example of the exploration of counter-role is described in Case 5, where Glen very frequently explored counter-roles within each session. Glen chose the roles of both the protagonist and antagonist to act out within the same story. For example, he would be Jack and the Giant in the story of *Jack and the Beanstalk*. Glen became the small, clever hero versus the huge, menacing giant. In exploring counter-roles, a pattern for Glen, he may have been attempting to find a balance by playing these opposites. In order for treatment to be considered successful, a patient may need to look from both sides. A patient able to explore and understand counter-roles can experience a balance in his or her everyday self. Through exploring counter-roles a patient can explore other forces. By exploring these other sides, the self can become whole again.

The therapist, adhering to this concept, noted when a patient was able to invoke a counter-role on his or her own. A child was never told to act out a counter-role, as all roles invoked were of the patient's choosing. All roles were explored completely on the patient's own initiative. These occurrences have been noted within each case. In some instances, because of the relative brevity of the treatment, the patients did not explore counter-roles, but very well may have if the dramatherapy sessions had been continued.

Reflecting upon the role-play

Most out-of-role reflecting and processing of the role-play was done during the final cool-down phase of each session. While the props and accessories were being put away or while the make-up was being removed, the reflective process occurred. After the dramatization ended, the therapist took the opportunity to discuss the role-playing as a means of gaining insight. The child was asked about a favorite part of the story or a favorite moment of the story. Sometimes the children volunteered much information and feedback regarding their dramatization. Some children said very little. Direct interpretations were never used with the children in order to maintain their sense of security, in their new-found form of self-expression. According to Winnicott (1971, p.117), 'interpretation in such circumstances annihilates the creativity of the patient and is traumatic in the sense of being against the maturational process.' This is one instance where the role method was modified. Once the child specified a favorite moment, the therapist would proceed to discuss that scene with a focus on the emotional qualities that had been expressed. To avoid bias, the therapist did not necessarily mention stress. The scenes or moments favored by the children were noted and later analyzed for meaning or significance. During the out-of-role reflective stage of the dramatherapy session, non-confrontational questions were used, such as 'I wonder what that was like for them [role] to have been [chased, gobbled, left...]?' or 'How did they [role] feel when such and such happened to them?' or 'What did you like best about that part of the story?' or 'Was there something that you didn't like?' All out-of-role reflections that pertained to the characters were done during the last few minutes of each session.

In-role reflections, which occurred during the dramatizations and are detailed within each case, were another means of gaining information. There are differences between out-of-role and in-role reflections. A child is better able to reach self-expression through an indirect and less threatening form of communication, such as dramatic play. By expressing themselves symbolically or metaphorically, children are free to let down their defenses. The dramatizations themselves often unleashed an energy in the children, which motivated them to reflect out-of-role. This was in part due to the shared experience of creating live drama.

Relating the fictional roles to everyday life

This step was modified by the researcher as being potentially too confrontational or direct for the children. The children's medical and psychological conditions were tenuous. The dramatherapy intervention was designed as short-term therapy at ten sessions per individual. Because of these factors the researcher decided not to relate the fiction to the child's reality, at least not with the child's direct participation. This breaks the fourth wall of the dramatic play and can damage a child's ability to suspend their disbelief. Interpretations can reverse the progress of such patients.

It was the therapist's job to relate the fictional roles enacted by the patients to their everyday life, unbeknown to the child. Because their everyday lives were dictated by chronic illness, the roles selected and created were related to the intrinsic nature and the emotional repercussions of their illness. The stress experienced by the fictional roles often relates to the stress experienced by the patients in everyday life. An example of this would be Case 3. Brandon would huff and puff with great frustration and anger while in the role of the Wolf in *The Three Little Pigs*. The stress and emotions expressed by the frustrated Wolf related to Brandon's own angst regarding his difficulty breathing. Relating the stress of the fictional roles to the stress in the patient's everyday life is therefore significant in determining whether or not there was a reduction in stress as a result of the dramatherapy treatment.

The children were made aware of the qualities and functions of their role through the reflection process. However, the therapist never interpreted the relation between the fictional role and everyday life unless the children discovered it themselves. The researcher felt that the children would benefit more if they felt free to express themselves through a playful and seemingly natural manner without the knowledge that they were actually communicating their own feelings regarding their illness. These were children who for the most part did not want to talk about their medical condition, let alone express their feelings about it. Also, because of the relatively short treatment time having been designed for ten sessions, it was deemed too soon to intrude on their story making.

Integrating roles to create a functional role system

As stated, some patients tended to stay with one role, while others explored several roles at once. The exploration of roles could easily change from session to session. The significance of how the various roles worked together, including any thematic considerations and patterning, was the work for the researcher as part of the overall analysis. Although some of the children became more verbal as the sessions progressed, any reference to the integration that may have occurred was done so in an informal way. There were clear shifts within the role system in many cases, while in other cases shifts were minimal. In Case 4, for example, Aaron played the role of the Wolf repeatedly. The only other two roles he invoked were very early on in the treatment and were both antagonists as well. His role selection was singularly focused and did not allow for integration. In Case 5, Glen played up to eight roles in any given session, which allowed for more of an integration based on the variety of qualities and functions he was able to explore. Any acknowledgment of the importance of both the positive and negative roles was done so by the acceptance by the therapist of any qualities expressed.

Social modeling

This suggests that once a client breaks unhealthy patterns for themselves, new models must be provided for the significant people in his or her life. A client allows for this positive internal change to have an effect on others, so that the people within one's social system can effectively learn to adjust and adapt to a healthier role system through social modeling.

Because of the relatively short length of the dramatherapy intervention, pattern making was established rather than pattern breaking. Any of the abusive or negative cyclical patterns that had emerged may have been explored more fully, if the treatment involved more sessions. Although other people within the child's social sphere had noticed some changes in the patient's behavior, how or if social modeling had occurred may have been simply too soon to tell (Landy 1993).

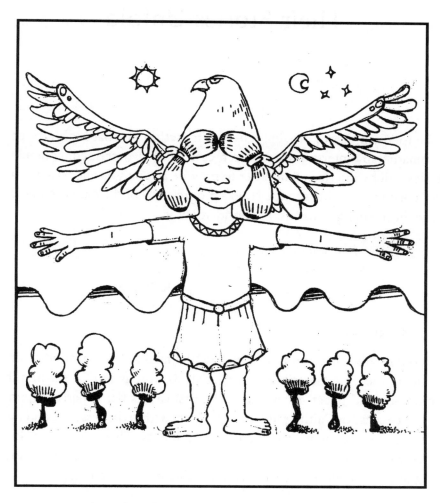

Figure 4.1 As the Bird, Caitlin was able to fly with a strength from within (illustration by Laurence Muleh 2001)

CHAPTER 4

Their Stories Unfold

The following cases provide selected transcriptions that highlight the dramatherapy intervention. As each case study is described, commentaries will be interjected in order to provide an analysis and as a means of reflecting insight as to the child's progress. All of the patients' names have been changed to ensure confidentiality.

> *All that is gold does not glitter,*
> *Not all those who wander are lost.*
> J.R.R. Tolkien

And So She Flew...

Each individual case study will include the medical background of the patient, the case description and analysis, discussion, a six-month follow-up and selected transcript. The first case is particularly inspirational because of Caitlin's dramatic progress within the sessions, and the marked improvement in her once grave illness. This is noted in her one-year follow-up. She was considered to be the most physically fragile of the children before the dramatherapy intervention.

Background

Caitlin is a 6-year-old girl diagnosed with severe pulmonary hypertension, BPD (broncho-pulmonary dysplasia), and developmental delay. She was delivered prematurely at 26 weeks gestational age, with a weight of less than two pounds. Hers is a severe condition which, until recently, could only be treated by a heart and lung transplant. She is, however, on a new drug treatment program which is experimental yet appears to be working. She has a Hickman catheter inserted in a vein behind her clavicle that delivers medication directly to her heart. The medications are contained in a brightly colored backpack that she wears every day. She takes nine medications including liquids and pills each day. These medications include prostacycline, lasix, digoxin, aldactone, and albuterol. Caitlin is on 24-hour oxygen. She wheels her oxygen tank around with her as tubes are gently secured into her nostrils. She's been on oxygen 24 hours a day since she was born.

Caitlin's condition is grave; when she gets a cold it becomes a major respiratory illness. She has shortness of breath, fevers, and bad infections, and she is often hospitalized. She frequently cries when needles are used to draw blood samples. Caitlin has a developmental speech impediment and delay. She has had episodes of falling down that occur with or without activity, yet denies any dizziness associated with falling. Caitlin has had bilateral hernia repair surgery (8/91) and cardiac catheterization procedures on several occasions (1/92, 10/93, 2/96). Most recently, Caitlin was hospitalized on 3/20/97, 5/29/97, and 6/26/97 for heart-related problems.

Caitlin's visual motor control and upper limb coordination is that of someone of 4 years/8 months. She is considered to be impulsive and distractible. She has difficulty defining simple words, and her ability to remain focused on a topic is poor. She is minimally expressive and moderately receptive with a language disorder. Caitlin has both speech and physical therapy twice weekly. She has attended this school/day hospital program for just over one year.

Description and Analysis

Session #1: Introduction

Caitlin was initially presented as a fragile, shy and timid girl who was curious about drama but seemed only minimally interested. This was indicated by her somewhat distracted behavior. She had very poor eye contact and her speech was nearly inaudible. The therapist had to ask her two to three times to repeat most of what she said and only at times could she even then be understood. Although Caitlin appeared as a bright and amiable child, her behavior was somewhat distant and her affect was flat. She never smiled or interacted with much emotion or expression. She seemed depressed. Although she was a pretty child with fashionable outfits, she was difficult to reach. She had had her illness her entire life; it was all that she knew. And although she could get around and maneuver her oxygen tank on wheels with apparent ease (her tank being on an apparatus over a foot taller than she), there was a sadness in her eyes. She appeared to be under stress because of her chronic medical condition. Caitlin was distractible and fidgety. She seemed difficult to connect with, at least at first.

Session #2: The Three Little Pigs

During the first dramatherapy session, she listened as the therapist told her the story she had selected, *The Three Little Pigs*. She listened with no particular facial expression. It seemed that she really wanted to look into the 'drama bag,' but was patient until the story ended. This was to become a ritual with Caitlin. As soon as the story ended she smiled and leaned toward the bag and awaited the therapist's approval. Then she rooted through the bag, delighted to find puppets, masks, hats, make-up, and costume accessories all at her disposal. As she explored the contents of the bag, the therapist asked Caitlin who she would like to be. She was told that she could select any person, animal, or thing from the story. She picked 'Mother.' As she continued to look at the drama items, she indicated an interest in the masks.

COMMENTARY 1

She already appeared to be wearing a mask, in the form of the oxygen tubes that wrapped around her face and into her nostrils. She focused on a pink, furry, soft pig mask for her role as 'Mother.' The therapist helped her to put it on, careful not to disturb her tubes, which were her life support. She now appeared to be wearing a mask over her own mask of tubes. It seemed a double form of distancing.

The use of the double masking provides a safe and distanced place from which Caitlin can begin her journey. Theatrically stylized accessories made available for use in therapy offer both safety and distance to the patient. Chronically ill children need to have a safe place from which to express themselves, because of the frailty of their condition.

When asked, she specifically selected the scene where the Pigs were in the brick house, as being her favorite part of the story. She directed the therapist to be the Wolf by using a Wolf puppet. So the Wolf huffed and puffed. 'Not by the hair of my chinny chin chin ...,' she said. The Wolf did not blow down the house, and Mother remained safe inside.

COMMENTARY 2

She was in the role of the Mother Pig in the scene where the Wolf is trying to get all three of her children. This is the scene where both the climax and conflict occur. She acted out the most stressful scene, yet in the safest way, as the Mother in the brick house. Mother is not in that particular scene in the original story. It may be that Mother's presence was needed. Caitlin then had to leave the therapy room to use the bathroom, which may be considered indicative of some anxiety. Interestingly, Caitlin only selected the most stressful scene of the story to act out. The Wolf's attempt to blow down the brick house, using his breath (oxygen) as his primary means, which in fact fails him, is similar to Caitlin's daily struggle to breathe, which is only made possible by her oxygen tanks and tubes. The Wolf's breath fails him and he dies. If it weren't for Caitlin's oxygen tanks, she would not be alive either. This was the first session for Caitlin and she did not want to act out that role directly, yet it did have an impact. She clearly needed to be in the role of Mother, who in this case actually was an integral part of 'saving the day.' Mother was in the brick home with the Pigs, unlike the original version, to help in their very survival. Caitlin adjusted the role of the Mother and gave her the function of protecting and nurturing her children. She was also in the role of helper.

It was over the first few sessions that the role of Mother was the most comfortable role for Caitlin to try. She selected the Mother from *The Three Little Pigs* (session 2) and then the Mother from *Little Red Riding Hood* (session 4).

COMMENTARY 3

The role of Mother is neither antagonist nor protagonist, but is the universal role of nurturer and a figure on whom others are dependent. Through this role Caitlin explored qualities of dependence, security and comfort. According to Landy's (1993) taxonomy, 'the conventional mother is moral, loving, caring and nurturing.' She is a survivor. Universally, the physical qualities of Mother include beauty, inner strength, and good health. Cognitively, the role of Mother is wise and knowing. This role which Caitlin had invoked had emotions that included loving, maternal, and life-producing qualities. Caitlin had chosen this powerful, yet comforting role to explore, not only because of its much needed qualities, but because of its very function. The 'good' Mother is a survivor, which is what Caitlin was fighting to be. Yet, she was so ill and so fragile that she needed the nurturing and protection of a mother figure. The role of Mother is the first role that Caitlin explored. The role of Mother is representational in style, since she represents reality in these two stories. The Mother of The Three Little Pigs *and of* Little Red Riding Hood *essentially directs her child/children with warnings as they venture into the world. In* The Three Little Pigs *Mother actually forces them to go against their will. In* Little Red Riding Hood *Mother tells her daughter to go through the woods to Grandmother's house. In both instances it is because of the mother that the children face great danger: the hungry Wolf. These moments in the stories are indicative of the issue of separation anxiety.*

Session #4: Little Red Riding Hood

It was during the fourth session that Caitlin explored the role of Mother, and developed what was to become her signature role. Up to this point, Caitlin had been minimally interactive and slightly distracted. After she selected and heard the story of *Little Red Riding Hood*, she spent some time simply setting up plastic/toy plates and cups upon a chair and the arms of the chair. She was stacking and balancing them.

COMMENTARY 4

This seemed to be reflective of her need for physical balance, as was indicated in the medical chart by her occasional loss of balance. Yet, this play indicated some resistance. She wasn't ready. She seemed to be avoiding her turn to act in the story.

Then she said, 'OK, ready. OK, ready, I'll be upstairs sleeping and you can call me.'

Mom/Caitlin:	Oh, Red Riding Hood. [*She calls in a singsong fashion.*]
Little Red/Therapist:	What?
Mom:	Can you go down into the woods for me? [*slightly inaudible*]
Little Red:	Mother? What? [*The staff explained that she not only has a speech impediment but also a thick Brooklyn accent.*]
Mom:	Go to the woods, 'cause your Grandmother is sick.
Little Red:	Grandmother is sick? Is there anything wrong?
Mom:	No. [*She says with a hint of avoidance.*]

COMMENTARY 5

The nurse explained that whenever anyone asks Caitlin about her oxygen tank or her illness, she would refer them to a nurse to answer further. She will simply say that nothing is wrong. Therefore, when she states that nothing is really wrong with Grandmother, she may be projecting her own avoidance. The therapist anticipates Caitlin's response regarding the issue of illness. As Caitlin avoids the issue, the therapist is careful not to question her any further.

Little Red/Therapist:	All right, yes, Mother. Would you like me to bring anything to Grandmother?
Mom/Caitlin:	Yes. Cookies and, umm, snacks.
Little Red:	Cookies and some snacks? [*The therapist has to repeat a lot of what she says to make sure she's been heard correctly.*]
Mom:	OK.
Little Red:	Should I go now?
Mom:	Yeah.
Little Red:	Bye, Mother.
Mom:	Bye.
Narrator/Therapist:	So Little Red went off into the woods [*whistling*]. I'm going to Grandmother's. I'm going to Grandmother's house [*singing*].

Then, as the story unfolds, Caitlin takes time to set up some animal puppets to be in the woods. She explains that the animals are there to help Little Red. As Little Red continues through the woods she sees the bird (puppet) that Caitlin is now wearing.

COMMENTARY 6

The therapist has a variety of puppets, masks, make-up and accessories available so that the patients can choose what is comfortable for them at any given point during the treatment process. Puppets are more distanced than masks, which are more distanced than make-up. Because a puppet is worn on the hand rather than on one's face, it is safer. Caitlin needs to feel this distance, in order to express herself through her newly invoked role of the Bird.

Little Red/Therapist:	Oh, here we are on the way to Grandmother's house. Oh, it's a bird! Birdie! [*she calls*] Little Birdie! I'm going to Grandmother's house, but listen, I'm a little worried because I ran into this Wolf, and he was talking to me and, I don't know, I'm afraid that maybe he might go there, too.
Bird/Caitlin:	That's OK. I will help you.
Little Red:	Will you help me? [*She nods.*] Thank you, Bird. Thank you for helping me out, so that I'm not scared. Will you go with me to my Grandmother's?
Bird:	Yeah.
Little Red:	But what if the Wolf's there?
Bird:	[*barely audible*] I will eat him.
Little Red:	You will? 'Cause I don't want the Wolf to eat me. Oh, thank you, Bird. You're the best friend a girl could have.
Bird:	Thank you.
Little Red:	Thank you so much, Birdie.
Bird:	Thank you.
Therapist:	[*whispered out of character as therapist*] Should we take any more animals or just take the bird?
Bird:	Just take the bird.

Little Red:	Come on, little Birdie, let's go to Grandmother's house. Here we go.
Therapist:	Now, do you want me to be Little Red all the way?
Caitlin:	Little Red.
Therapist:	OK, ummm, we'll pretend the Wolf is in the chair.
Little Red:	Grandmother, Grandmother, what big eyes you have.
Wolf/Therapist:	The better to see you with, my dear.
Little Red:	Grandmother, I would like you to meet my friend, the little Bird. [*To Bird*] This is my Grandmother, ohhh! [*Bird eats Grandmother*] what did you do to my Grandmother?
Bird:	I ate him. He was the Wolf.
Little Red:	Ohhhh! Ohhhh! Thank you, Bird!
Bird:	You're welcome.
Little Red:	Because if you hadn't done that, then the Grandmother, the Wolf, might have gobbled me up. Wait, where's Grandmother?
Bird:	She's home.
Little Red:	Oh, thank you Bird. How can I ever repay you? Is there anything I can do?
Bird:	I can take you back home.
Little Red:	Yes, please take me back home. It is where I really want to be. Can I follow you?
Bird:	Yes.
Little Red:	Thank you, Bird.
Bird:	Thanks.
Little Red:	Let's see if Mom is home. [*calls*] Mom? Where's my Mom?
Bird:	I think she's upstairs taking a shower.
Little Red:	Taking a shower? Well when she comes downstairs, I'm going to tell my Mom that you were the best Bird that a girl could ever have. The nicest Bird…why you saved my life. You saved me from the wicked Wolf 'cause, you

know what? He was pretending to be Grandmother and I didn't even know. How did you know?

Bird: Because.

Little Red: That was so nice of you. How can I ever repay you?

Bird: Thank everyone.

Little Red: What?

Bird: Thank everyone.

Little Red: OK. I'd like to thank you, my favorite Bird. And I would like to thank everyone who helped to save my life so that the Wolf wouldn't get me 'cause that wouldn't have been very nice. Thank you so much, Bird, bye…

Bird: Bye. Before we go can we have some food and put out the plates?

As the session concludes, the Bird character proceeds to make 'macaroni and cheese with fruit punch for everyone.' A celebration unfolds and all of the woodland animals are invited. She appeared to be the Mother as she cooked, but she said that she was still the Bird and she was to become the Bird from that day on, for every session to come.

COMMENTARY 7

Caitlin had begun her exploration of self during the first few sessions as Mother, but during session 4 this transformed into the role of the Bird. The actual puppet that she used was a toucan with a large, brightly colored beak, substantial enough for eating wolves, with one eye replaced by a button due to past battles. A bird is generally considered to be small and somewhat fragile, as is Caitlin. Her need for physical balance may be explored by the bird's grace and ability to fly. The bird's large beak may be indicative of her struggle with her severe speech impediment. Up to this point she has not been particularly verbal, probably because when she does speak it is often inaudible. Yet, she is able to express much through the role playing. According to Handoo (1990), animals in the real world are of two types:

small/weak = unwise = defeat;
big/strong = wise = victory.

Whereas animals in folklore are:

small/weak = wise = victory;
big/strong = unwise = defeat.

Caitlin's role of the Bird is the small/weak, as she actually is physically, which equals wisdom and a successful victory over the big, strong, yet unwise and consequently defeated, Wolf of the story. As opposed to the real world, 'in folklore, particularly narrative folklore, this attitude is inverted, and small, physically weak animals or birds are essentially victorious in their tasks and struggles against them' (Handoo 1990, p.7). Caitlin was born prematurely and is very small for her age. Her chronic heart condition and dependency on oxygen and IV medication make her physically weak. Caitlin developed this character of the Bird that wasn't even presented in the original storytelling. The animal symbolizes processes of both projection and internalization. This further promotes the concept that the role selects the player (Landy 1993).

The bird is considered to be 'the quest of the mind for the heights. It can signify the mind trapped in a primitive, subhuman condition. It rises from the earth to the sky above, like the shift from the body to mind; transcending bare, physical existence' (Chetwynd 1982, p.50). Caitlin's physical restrictions include the 24-hour IV housed in her backpack and entering her chest into her heart, and the equally restrictive 24-hour oxygen tank that she wheels around on a metal frame almost twice her height allowing air to enter through her nostrils. Because of these restraints, she cannot run, skip, or jump rope like other children. As the Bird, however, she could fly.

The role of the bird can be defined according to Landy (1993) by considering its qualities. Physically, the bird that Caitlin created is strong and healthy, unlike herself, who is physically weak and sickly. Cognitively, the bird is wise and all-knowing to the point of foreshadowing events to come. Morally, the role of the bird is innocent, much like Caitlin herself. Yet, this role is neither the role of the victim or the victimizer. The bird comes to the aid of the victim, and watches over the victim of each story as would a guardian angel.

The function of this original role that Caitlin invoked repeatedly throughout the dramatherapy sessions was to help the poor protagonist in an almost spiritual manner. The style of the Bird was presentational in that it was overdistanced and lacking in overt emotions. There was not an abundance of affect. Caitlin was able to be reflective through the role of the Bird. She was able to reflect on the protagonist's dilemmas as they mirrored her own. Once Caitlin designed this role, which was very early on during the third session, she continued in just this one role.

Caitlin needed to be in the role of the Bird, rather than explore any other roles, because it was a secure, yet effective role for her. If the dramatherapy treatment had continued after the ten scheduled sessions, she may have eventually invoked new roles or sub-roles. Once a child has fully explored a personally significant role, he or she eventually tries on new roles, having satisfied initial needs. This does not suggest that he or she will not return to the original and secure role; this will often happen. However, in Caitlin's case, if the ten sessions are indicative, then future sessions would suggest further growth through a wider role repertoire.

The quality, function, and style of the Bird presented Caitlin an opportunity to be what she wanted and to achieve what she needed to achieve. As the Bird, Caitlin was able to soar with strength, knowing all would be well once the brutal force was defeated. Caitlin took on a healthy and free role armed with the knowledge that obstacles could be destroyed. This relates to Caitlin's everyday life, in that she is fighting for her health in an attempt to be free. The Bird is Caitlin's preferred choice of roles. The type of this role is that of 'helper.' The qualities of the role of helper appear as the 'unselfish, supportive…good friend' (Landy 1993). Caitlin's portrayal of the helper includes additional qualities, such as an inner knowledge and a genuine concern.

Having created the role of Bird in the story of Little Red Riding Hood, *Caitlin applied the qualities of the role of helper to the Bird, even being referred to as 'the best friend a girl could ever have' by the therapist in the role of Little Red. According to Landy (1993, p.197), the function of the helper is 'to move the hero or protagonist further along his path or to rescue another from difficult circumstances, remaining loyal throughout the many twists and turns of the journey.' The function of the helper was adhered to as the Bird helped Little Red along the literal path and rescued her from the Wolf by devouring him. She was loyal and unselfish in her ability to save lives. Caitlin is facing a life-threatening illness. The related symbol for the bird is the volatile element: air, gases and steam (Chetwynd 1982), which is Caitlin's lifeline (oxygen from the tank). It is the air within the story that allows the bird to fly free.*

Session #5: The Three Little Pigs

Caitlin hadn't been to therapy in over a week because of the school's vacation. All the children had been working on a special art/T-shirt project that afternoon. The staff stated for the therapist to work with whoever was willing to go at that time. Caitlin had just finished her project and volunteered to go for drama. She was eager and willing to attend. Up until this point she had seemed slightly distracted and minimally interactive. She was now much more interactive and presented more of an ease that had come over her. It appeared as though a transformation may have been evolving. She remembered the story that had been done during the last session that was over a week ago, without hesitation. Caitlin selected the story of *The Three Little Pigs* for this fifth session. She appeared eager. Since she had done this story during a previous session, she was given the choice of the therapist's telling her the story again or not; she wanted to hear the story.

During this session she was more verbal and attentive. As soon as the story was over, she smiled to get the therapist's approval for her to open the drama bag. 'Now can I open it?' she asked. She knew as soon as the story was over she was free to explore the bag of 'goodies.' She selected the bird puppet as her favorite character to enact. There was no mention of a bird in the story, but she had connected with this character from the last session. The Bird would help all the Pigs in the story.

She began by suggesting that the first Pig needed to buy bricks, so 'when the Wolf comes, it will work.' She continued to offer her help in building the house when the lazy Pig complained that it would be too much work. She told the Pig where to get bricks. But the Pig did not heed the Bird's advice or warnings. Then the second Pig came along, and once again the Bird tried to suggest bricks for the Pig to use in building his house. But the Pig did not listen. It is the third Pig who takes the Bird's advice and buys bricks from the Old Man. The Bird actually told the Old Man that he wanted bricks and then, without complaint, proceeded to help the Pig build his house of bricks.

Meanwhile, the Wolf made his rounds blowing down the straw and stick houses, as the Bird continued to advise them where to run. In fact, they followed the Bird into the safety of the brick house. The older Pig explained how he took the Bird's advice and how the Bird helped him to build the house. When the Wolf arrived, the Bird was the one to suggest putting the bubbling pot under the chimney.

COMMENTARY 8

The Bird was overlapping into the smart Pig's role of being responsible for saving their lives. This moment in the story, as well as the last session's moment of the Bird actually eating the Wolf, are both indicative of the issue of fear of bodily harm or death. If the Bird does not act quickly, under pressure, to kill the Wolf, then lives will be lost. In this scenario, the Wolf wants to devour the Pigs, but the Bird saves their lives.

The minute the story was over, Caitlin asked to use the bathroom. This was the exact moment when she enacted this same story during the first session that Caitlin had to use the bathroom before. This issue of fear of bodily harm or death may have been anxiety-provoking for her.

She took a short break. When she returned, with a few minutes left in the session, an informal interview ensued, with the use of the tape recorder which recorded all sessions.

Therapist:	This is Ms Carol and Caitlin having drama together. We just finished acting out a story. Now, Caitlin would like to say hello.
Caitlin:	Hello.
Therapist:	Caitlin, can you tell us what story we just did?
Caitlin:	*The Three Little Pigs.*
Therapist:	And can you tell us, Caitlin, what character you got to be?
Caitlin:	The Bird.
Therapist:	And how did you get to be a bird? Did you become the bird?
Caitlin:	Yes.
Therapist:	And did you have a puppet to help you?
Caitlin:	Yes.
Therapist:	And can you tell everyone where you went for vacation?
Caitlin:	To the beach.

COMMENTARY 9

Rather than directly interpreting or investigating the dramatherapy process with Caitlin, the therapist changes the subject to something seemingly comfortable for the patient, that being vacation. Discussing a welcoming topic can reduce any inhibitions which were forming, as were indicated by her single-word answers.

Therapist:	And tell us what you think about the beach.
Caitlin:	Going on the rides.
Therapist:	Oh, you got to go on the rides?
Caitlin:	Yes.
Therapist:	And did you get to go in the water?
Caitlin:	Yes.
Therapist:	What is your favorite part? The water, the sand or the rides?
Caitlin:	Lots of them.
Therapist:	Lots of rides? Can you tell everyone how old you are?
Caitlin:	Six.
Therapist:	And what school do you go to, Caitlin?
Caitlin:	[*She names the school*]
Therapist:	And can you please tell us, what it is about [the school] that you like?
Caitlin:	At the hospital.
Therapist:	You like that it's at the hospital?
Caitlin:	Yes.
Therapist:	What's something about [the school] that you don't like. Is there anything?
Caitlin:	I like everything.
Therapist:	Caitlin says that she likes everything about [the school]. And tell us what you think about doing drama with Ms Carol?
Caitlin:	It's pretty fun.
Therapist:	It's pretty fun. And would you recommend it to your friends?
Caitlin:	Yes.
Therapist:	And what is your favorite story of all time that was done?
Caitlin:	*The Three Little Pigs.*

Therapist:	*The Three Little Pigs.* And *The Three Little Pigs* is the story that we did for today. All right, let's say goodbye to our recorder, please. Caitlin, would you like to say goodbye?
Caitlin:	Bye.
Therapist:	Bye. We hope to see you again. Is there something else you would like to add.
Caitlin:	Add?
Therapist:	Is there anything you would like to say?
Caitlin:	Umm, oh yeah. We went to the uh…we went into the hotel and spent a lot of money.
Therapist:	You went to the hotel and it cost a lot of money. Those hotels do cost a lot of money. But was that fun for you?
Caitlin:	Yes.
Therapist:	Oh, and tell everyone about your new haircut.
Caitlin:	My Mom fixed the haircut.
Therapist:	Caitlin has a brand new haircut. It's a nice new style. Can you tell us about what this is [*gesture towards oxygen tank*]? The tank that's here, what is that?
Caitlin:	A tank.
Therapist:	And what is the tank for?
Caitlin:	I don't know [*she says reluctantly*].

COMMENTARY 10

Having established that the conversation was about to end, the therapist then asked more direct questions regarding Caitlin's medical apparatus. Her resistance and defensiveness regarding these issues were apparent.

Therapist:	We don't know, but it's on wheels and Caitlin gets to ride on it, it helps her scoot along on wheels a little faster. Is that right?
Caitlin:	Yeah, I guess so.
Therapist:	Do you like this tank?
Caitlin:	Yeah.

Therapist:	And do you want to tell us what this tube is for? We're not sure what this is for.
Caitlin:	I don't know [*she says dejectedly*].
Therapist:	Well, then we don't have to tell what it is. Can you tell me who's on your backpack? I see Pocahontas. [*Pause*] So, anyway, it's time to turn off the tape and then we'll play back our story. So let's say goodbye for now.
Caitlin:	Goodbye.

COMMENTARY 11

This informal interview explored Caitlin's ability to process and verbalize some of her thoughts and feelings. Caitlin is minimally verbal, and sometimes has difficulty formulating sentences or responses that are appropriate. Her language disorder warrants speech therapy twice weekly. Caitlin has developmental speech delay with minimal expressiveness and moderate receptiveness. Her resistance and awkwardness in discussing her intrusive and highly visible medical equipment has been verified and confirmed by her primary nurse. She doesn't want to talk about it. As many of the patients, she has been referred to by the Director of Psychology, Dr K (personal communication, June 14 1997) as being 'a child who is experiencing loss and pain, yet can't verbalize it. This is why an alternate form of therapy, such as dramatherapy, is so important for these kids.'

Session #6: Little Red Riding Hood

During the next session, Caitlin again is eager to attend. Her countenance is noticeably more positive. She seems vibrant. She remembers the story that had been done during the session before. She is smiling more. She selects the story of 'Little Red.' As she listens to the story, she is more attentive. She has better eye contact and is not as fidgety or distracted as in the early sessions.

Therapist:	If you could be anyone in the story, who would you be?
Caitlin:	[*She pulls the bird puppet out of the bag in response.*]
Therapist:	What will the Bird do in *Little Red Riding Hood*?
Caitlin:	To help out.
Therapist:	That's a good idea. What can you do to help?

Caitlin:	Help her from the Wolf.
Therapist:	The Bird can help Little Red Riding Hood from the Wolf. He could warn her or help her. What's another good idea?
Caitlin:	He can eat him up.
Therapist:	Little Red needs some help, doesn't she?

COMMENTARY 12

Over these weeks, Caitlin has increased the story line that is acted out, from one scene, to most of the story, to the entire story. This indicated less distractibility, and more focus and interaction. She proceeded to help by warning the protagonist, rescuing and saving their lives. The role of the Bird has become and will continue to be Caitlin's preferred role. 'The invocation of the role...is a calling into being of that part of the person that will inspire a creative search for meaning. [This] invocation usually proceeds unconsciously' (Landy 1993, p.47). The invocation is unconscious for Caitlin, as is the meaning. Yet, the power of the unconscious to heal is at work. The therapist allows the patient to select any role that she chooses. It is imperative that the therapist doesn't select or suggest a role for her. The patient's invoking of a role is indicative of her unconscious needs. If the patient needs to expand their role repertoire they will do it at their own pace and only once they have explored the necessary significance of a selected role. Not only has Caitlin created her own role, but consequently has added her own story line.

The Bird (Caitlin) warns Little Red (Therapist) about the Wolf's true motivation while in the woods. When Little Red arrives at Grandmother's house, the little Bird accompanies her.

Little Red / Therapist:	[*Knocks on door.*]
Wolf / Therapist:	[*In Grandmother's voice*] Come in...
Little Red:	[*Enters, looks at Grandmother*] Grandmother, look...hey, I have to talk to my friend. [*To Bird*] Grandmother is over in that bed but she sure doesn't look like herself?
Bird / Caitlin:	It's the Wolf.
Little Red:	Ohh, Ohh!
Bird:	He ate Grandmother up.

Little Red:	Ohh, the Wolf ate up Grandmother and now he's in bed!? [*To Grandmother/Wolf*] I'll be right there. [*To Bird*] What should I do?
Bird:	I can help you.
Little Red:	How?
Bird:	I can eat him.
Little Red:	You can eat the Wolf? OK, come with me. [*To Grandmother/Wolf*] Grandmother, what big eyes you have.
Wolf:	The better to see you with, my dear.
Little Red:	Grandmother, what big ears you have.
Wolf:	The better to hear you with, my dear.
Little Red:	Grandmother [*Bird enters*].
Bird:	Watch this [*Bird flies over*].
Narrator/Therapist:	And the Bird flew over to the mean old Wolf dressed like Grandmother.
Wolf:	Hey! [*Growls*]
Narrator/Therapist:	And the Wolf tried to eat the Bird. But the Bird ate the Wolf.
Little Red:	Oohh, did you gobble the Wolf?
Bird:	[*Nods*]
Little Red:	Thank you! Ooh, otherwise he would've gobbled me. Wait, where is Grandmother?
Bird:	She's out.
Little Red:	There she is. Is she out?
Bird:	[*Nods*]
Little Red:	Grandmother is fine. Bird, you have saved the day. If you hadn't come in when you did and gobbled up the Wolf, he would've gobbled me up. That was so nice of you.
Bird:	Thank you.
Little Red:	Well, thank you. Would you like to come live with myself and my Mother? Let's go to my house and tell

Mother what happened. [*So they go to visit Mother and process what had happened.*]

Mother / Therapist: I must thank you for saving my daughter. Even though you're a small little Bird you really saved the day. How did you do it?

Bird: I talked.

Mother: What?

Bird: I liked to talk to her.

Mother: You attacked?

COMMENTARY 13

It is difficult understanding Caitlin due to her speech impediment. When she said 'talk,' it sounded like 'attack.' She states that 'talking' is how she saved the day, yet her own ability to talk is often inaudible. The Bird actually did attack the Wolf, yet Caitlin was saying 'talk.' It was actually the bird's talking and foreshadowing that proved to be helpful. Caitlin's insight into the pending threat, which she verbalized, was in fact through talking. Caitlin's own difficulty with being understood is frustrating for her. Whenever someone has to repeatedly ask 'what?' Caitlin may be feeling a personal attack.

Bird / Caitlin: I talked to her.

Mother / Therapist: And you knew she needed help. I told her not to talk to strangers. How did this happen?

Bird: Today.

Mother: Today.

When asked if she was afraid of the Wolf, she was ambivalent in her answer, she nodded yes, then no, then yes. Finally, she shook her puppet head no, yes, then no.

Mother / Therapist: Do you have a name?

Bird / Caitlin: [*No response*]

Mother: Are you a boy bird or a girl bird?

Bird: Boy [she answers with no hesitation].

Mother:	Can you describe the Bird?
Bird:	Like a parrot.
Mother:	Are you nice?
Bird:	Yes.

COMMENTARY 14

The therapist explores some in-role questioning, but doesn't gain much information because of the patient's minimal responses and inability to verbalize extensively. Dramatherapy with chronically ill children is not based on their ability to verbalize, but is rooted in images, symbolism and the action of the stories as they relate to pertinent issues. Minimally verbal patients will simply not use dialogue as their primary mode of communication, which is why dramatherapy can be so useful with these children.

Caitlin continues in the role of the Bird. She is neither protagonist nor antagonist. She is in an auxiliary role. It is certainly a much safer role than any other. Yet, it is significant because she becomes the guiding light. She has all the answers. In addition to her verbal warnings and advice, she actually kills the Wolf by devouring him. She conquers the antagonist with no help from the rather naive and innocent Little Red. She is battling the threat of death and winning. In fact 'in mythology, the dead soul may be seen as a bird. The bird may also symbolize the very beginning of life. In this way the symbol of the bird may contain the bird motif and also, the death motif. When the bird motif turns up in psychotherapy, it is important to bear in mind the theme of birth and the theme of death' (Brun et al. 1993, p.123). Caitlin has been facing death since her premature birth with a life-threatening illness. It appears as though she is able to fight death symbolically through the dramatization of fairy tales.

By playing the role of the Bird, Caitlin is symbolically exploring birth and death. Landy (1993) discusses the idea of the counter-role within the role method. The counter-role is another side of a main role. There needs to be a balance in role selection and role playing. A client needs self-expression by exploring different angles. The therapist needs to observe any indication of the exploration of counter-roles over the course of the sessions, which can suggest a tendency towards balance – an integral part of the treatment. If a patient expresses him- or herself from a different side of one role, this can provide an achievement of balance in his or her own everyday life. Hopefully, the client can progress towards this goal, in order to achieve successful treatment according to the role method. By actively and repeatedly acting out the role of the Bird, Caitlin is actually exploring paradoxi-

cal qualities within the role of the Bird, rather than counter-roles. The Bird symbolizes birth and death. These qualities create an ambivalence within the role of the Bird. One of the goals of treatment is to help Caitlin to live within this apparent ambivalence.

The significance of death in these selected fairy tales is not coincidental. In Little Red Riding Hood, *death is in the form of a carnivore, which can be seen as a threat to a child's body. Since Caitlin lives with this threat every day, it was necessary for her to distance herself from this issue. She did so by distancing herself from the role of the Wolf and Little Red in the story, and by taking on the role of 'the Bird.' This role, which she created, didn't exist in the original story. This further emphasizes Caitlin's need for safety and distance from the issue of death. The Bird ate the adversary (Wolf) in order to save and protect the protagonist (Little Red). The Bird actually eats the Wolf and as a result, the protagonist achieves success. This is due to the Bird's actions, which occur, as in other fairy tales, only at the very last moment. In order to progress, one must take risks with no guarantee (Heuscher 1974). Just as the Bird symbolizes birth and death, the 'fairy tale experiences the origins of life and death as one. No rational foresight can cushion the leap into apparent nothingness which character- izes the existential crisis. Intellectual understanding only accentuates this paradox' (Heuscher 1974, p.62). Such is this case of a 6-year-old child who is struggling with a body that is failing her and a mind that cannot comprehend her precarious situation.*

Session #7: Hansel and Gretel

Caitlin became more verbal and she laughed for the first time as she relayed an earlier unrelated incident. She selected the story of *Hansel and Gretel* for the first time and commented on how she would be able to look in the bag when the story was over. 'Then I can look in the bag,' she said, smiling. Once again, she assumed the role of the Bird, with the use of the hand puppet. This story actually has a bird in it. When asked, she said that her favorite part of the story was when the parents talked about taking the children to the woods to abandon them: 'When they talk about taking the children away,' she said, 'when the children couldn't sleep.'

COMMENTARY 15

> *This is indicative of separation anxiety, as well as a fear of loss of control. It is during this scene that Hansel and Gretel are threatened by abandonment and separation from their parents. This feeling of isolation and solitude has replaced their former existence (Mallet 1984).*

She continued on to explain that the Bird would help the children. 'The other bird ate the bread crumbs,' she said, as she clearly differentiated her role as the helpful bird from the role of the destructive bird. According to Heuscher (1974):

> The dove represents an animal which can separate itself from the house by long distance, without forgetting from where it came. Invisible to parents in this ethereal force that surrounds the child like a helpful spirit (like a good fairy or the guardian angel). It appears during Hansel and Gretel's moments of despair in the woods, when the path is lost. It is as if the young child, emerging out of his earlier world (which is one of unity with mother) would certainly get lost in the dark forest of life with its voracious animals, if it were not for this helpful, spiritual force which comes to his assistance whenever the need is greatest. (p. 116)

Caitlin had taken on this role of the ethereal force as the role of the Bird developed further. This recurrence of life vs. death was forming a pattern. It was reflective of how 'delicate' this child's condition was.

As in earlier sessions, Caitlin continued to guide, warn, and foreshadow the harmful events as they unfolded. When the Witch turned evil, the Bird actually hid in the drama bag, indicating fear. There was an evolution of the adversaries within the stories as Caitlin explored them from session to session. She was ambivalent regarding the Bird's fear of the Wolf, which up to this point had been the only antagonist presented in the selected tales. Until session 7 she had only selected stories with a Wolf, including *The Three Little Pigs, Little Red Riding Hood*, and *The Gingerbread Man*. Many of the children, including Caitlin, referred to the Fox as a Wolf in *The Gingerbread Man*.

The Witch is a more developed ogre than the Wolf. The Witch eventually tells the protagonist exactly how she plans to plump up Hansel, bake and eat him. She is not as primitive as the Wolf, rather appearing to be more calculating and threatening. The Witch is more human, therefore less distanced. A Wolf is a wild animal expected to attack his prey. A Witch living in an ever-so-tempting gingerbread house is a visibly cruel, supernatural being with a human's brain and ability to think through her horrific plan. Witches are identified with all that is evil. The Witch is a significant and magical being, having been part of every known culture since the beginning of time and being clearly associated with death. Caitlin's decision to battle the Witch is a progression indicating her willingness to face greater obstacles.

The story of *Hansel and Gretel* itself is a much more complex tale than the stories she had explored in previous sessions. Consequently, she increased her dramatic interactions. Much more verbal during the sessions, the role of the Bird was becoming more insightful in her communication. She now continued to act out the entire story, as opposed to a single scene. She used complete sentences now.

Just before they meet the Witch, the Bird warns Gretel, 'She is going to put your brother in a cage…after lunch she's going to do it.' The protagonists pay no attention to the Bird's warning and the story unfolds as was told. 'You can push her into the fireplace,' suggests the Bird, when the children are feeling helpless. So, together, the Bird and Gretel push the Witch into the fireplace [oven]. During the processing done within character at the conclusion of the story, the Bird explains that the children hadn't listened to the Bird, and that she had tried to tell them. Once again it is the innocence and naivety of the protagonists that almost demand the spiritual force of the Bird.

During Caitlin's last three sessions, she continued in her role of the Bird. Now she focused on what was to be the most significant story, *Jack and the Beanstalk*.

Session #8: Jack and the Beanstalk

COMMENTARY 16

Jack and the Beanstalk *is considered to be one of the world's best-known and most-loved fairy tales (Jones 1995). The most familiar version was written in 1807, but the first story resembling* Jack and the Beanstalk *can be traced to 1730 and was entitled* Enchantment Demonstrated in the Story of Jack Spriggins and the Enchanted Bean. *It was actually designed as a skit, rather than as a verbal story (Opie 1974). This suggests that this story is over 270 years old.*

This magical tale has been traced to primitive myths and biblical tales. In the oldest of these tales, a poor man plants a magic bean and it grows into a tree that reaches to heaven. It is the relationship between earth and the world above the sky that is the root of the story. 'The belief that there is, could be, or ought to be, a means of ascending to a land in the sky is, of course, as old or older than Jacob's Ladder and the Tower of Babel' (Opie 1974). This celestial inference conjugates the symbolism of the bird and his ability to reach the sky.

All the stories told by the therapist, including Jack and the Beanstalk, *begin with, 'Once upon a time and very far away.' This classical time frame provides needed distance. As the story then unfolds, the beanstalk will take the Bird even higher than in the previous stories. As a bird in this story, Caitlin is able to soar up to the heavens unencumbered by invasive tubes, IVs, and oxygen tubes. Caitlin, with her life-threatening illness, is able to fly up to heaven in the role of the Bird. It is through* Jack and the Beanstalk *that Caitlin is able to go to the heavens repeatedly and then return to the safety of her home on earth, each time with various forms of gold.*

After hearing the story as told by the therapist, Caitlin was asked what her favorite part was. She replied, 'When they took the gold.' During the session, which was the first time she acted through this story, Caitlin (as the Bird) and the therapist (as Jack) took the gold, the hen that laid the golden eggs, and the golden harp, all at once.

COMMENTARY 17

In doing this, she reduced the tension and stress, which would have occurred when Jack and the Bird repeat the visit to the Giant's castle three times, as in the original story. Gold is considered to be of the highest value, 'the enduring essence of life' (Chetwynd 1982, p.177). The gold that is retrieved from the Giant's castle is representative of spirituality, whereas the gold coins represent a material value and the gold eggs suggest life's forces. 'It is the golden harp, however, that represented the eternally creative gold that revealed its value only in the ability of the owner to play the instrument' (Heuscher 1974, p.369). Caitlin's direct verbalization indicating her preference for this part of the story is, therefore, as if she is trying re-

peatedly to preserve her very essence through taking the gold objects and escaping with her life both figuratively and literally.

The role of the Bird had evolved over the weeks. The Bird was portrayed as the helper, foreshadowing and directing the other character (roles) as to what to do. Her role had developed into an even more integral and pivotal part of the story. She had even progressed in her ability to face fear. Having successfully battled the Wolf and the Witch in previous sessions, Caitlin now faced the most difficult obstacle, that of the Giant. She is so fearful of the Giant that the bird puppet she maneuvers actually hides from the Giant under the office table each time he cries out, 'Fee, fi, fo, fum.'

There is a moment of fear that appears in Caitlin's eyes when the Giant awakes. In order to minimize or manage the fear, the therapist creates a very stylized and distant Giant through the role playing. The role of the Giant doesn't directly acknowledge the Bird's presence in any way so as to avoid any direct feelings of threat. Also, the Giant is portrayed as being very slow and unaware, so that Caitlin in the role of the Bird has some feeling of control over this potentially scary situation.

The Giant is a type of beast. According to Landy (1993), qualities of the beast are 'characterized by extremely unattractive looks in face and body, sometimes extending to a moral and/or spiritual quality. The beast is the role of the ugly one.' Giants are characterized by their size. More significantly, in reference to this particular case is the function of the beast 'to frighten and terrify. On a more psychological level, the beast reveals the shadowy, dark side of human nature' (Landy 1993, p.176). Caitlin was confronting the beast, more specifically battling a Giant. Caitlin was not simply stealing the Giant's treasures, but by doing so was saving her own life. According to Chetwynd:

> *[Beasts] personify the tremendous force of the unconscious, usually in its negative, destructive aspect. Views, discoveries, and visions that are larger than life, and can tear a man's psyche to pieces may all take the form of giants (i.e. experiences which can't be formulated properly and may be very destructive). (Chetwynd 1982, p.169)*

An example of this is a 6-year-old girl such as Caitlin who has a life-threatening illness exacerbated by repeated surgeries and daily invasive procedures. This is the 'Giant' that she has to face, which cannot be 'formulated properly.' Giants are merciless and irrational. They can be ruthless and without reason, just as Caitlin's illness may appear to be. Both are larger than life. Caitlin doesn't actually play the role of the Giant; she acknowledges its dark existence as an opposing force. It is a counter-role she battles against, in order to find resolution. If the Giant wins, Jack and the Bird will be devoured. This is what they face to obtain the gold. Yet, they face it together.

Session #9: Jack and the Beanstalk

Once again Caitlin selected the story of *Jack and the Beanstalk* and the role of the Bird. During the following scene Caitlin incorporated her medical apparatus into the story. While Jack (therapist) and the Bird (Caitlin) were sleeping, the beanstalk grew from the magic beans.

Narrator / Therapist:	And while they were sleeping, outside of the window, a beanstalk grew. It grew taller and taller through the clouds, and when Jack woke up...
Jack / Therapist:	[*Yawns and stretches*] Where's my little Bird? Good morning.
Bird / Caitlin:	Morning.
Jack:	Oh, my gosh. Mom was so mad at us. We're in trouble, aren't we? Why did you tell me to buy beans?
Bird:	They're magic.
Jack:	Now we're in big trouble.
Bird:	No, we won't.
Jack:	What?
Bird:	We can get the money and we can get the gold.
Jack:	What are you talking about? Where are we going to find gold?
Bird:	The beanstalk.
Jack:	What beanstalk?
Bird:	That one [*points toward oxygen tank*].
Jack:	There's a beanstalk? Oohh, look! There is a beanstalk! Should we climb it?
Bird:	Yes.
Jack:	Do you want to go, too?
Bird:	Yes.

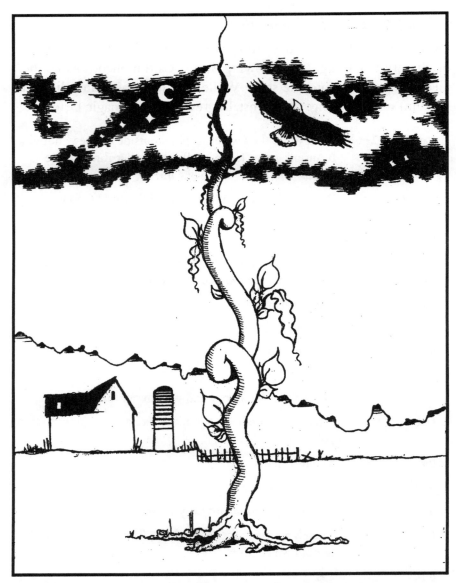

Figure 4.2 Soaring to great heights, Caitlin, as the Bird, reached for the heavens (illustration by Laurence Muleh 2001)

Jack:	Should we tell Mom?

Jack: Should we tell Mom?

Bird: [*Shakes her head no.*]

Jack: [*Whispers*] No, no, let's go.

Narrator/Therapist: So little Jack and the Bird went over to the beanstalk. [*The therapist and Caitlin both crossed over to the oxygen tank, which was the closest thing to a beanstalk in the small office. As they climbed, they pretended the oxygen tank was the beanstalk.*] And they climbed and climbed and climbed and then they climbed and climbed to the very top. Ooh, look, it's a castle…

During this session, Caitlin incorporated her towering oxygen tank and its five-foot stand as the beanstalk itself. The Bird (Caitlin) and Jack (therapist) pretended to climb up the oxygen stand apparatus whenever they journeyed from earth to the heavens.

COMMENTARY 18

The therapist was careful to follow Caitlin's lead in climbing up the oxygen tank, rather than directing her to do so. The patients must make discoveries for themselves in order for healing to occur. The beanstalk is what allows the Bird and Jack to go up to the castle in the sky, to explore their destiny. The Bird can't seem to fly up there without the beanstalk. Caitlin depends on her oxygen tank as a life support system, just as the beanstalk is necessary for the life of the story. However, the beanstalk, as is projected into the oxygen tank/stand, turns out to be the catalyst for the Giant's demise. When the Bird and Jack chop down the beanstalk, the Giant dies. Without Caitlin's towering oxygen stand, she couldn't survive. As Caitlin, in the role of the Bird, chopped down the beanstalk/oxygen stand she may have been projecting her own desire to get rid of this appendage.

As Caitlin reflected on the story after it was dramatized, she commented, with pride, on how the Bird helped to chop down the beanstalk. She stated that 'we did it together…we chopped it.' Then, she referred to Jack as being the Bird's brother.

COMMENTARY 19

Caitlin didn't feel comfortable being in the central role of the protagonist. But as the Bird she had more autonomy and less direct confrontation. However, as Jack's brother a bond and a closeness had been formed as she stepped closer to her fears.

Over the last three sessions she had transformed further. Caitlin's behavior changed drastically since the first few dramatherapy sessions, becoming more interactive with the therapist on a conversational level, and through her role-playing. From being only able to act out a scene from a story, she progressed to acting out the entire story from beginning to end. Her eye contact became focused and attentive; she no longer looked down or away. Her smile and overall positive attitude were a major change from when she first presented herself as a reserved, inhibited, fidgety and inattentive little girl. Her ability to focus and express herself in a more relaxed fashion were apparent. It was as if her newfound ability to fly like the Bird literally lifted her spirits. Her stress appeared to be greatly reduced.

Caitlin proceeded to explore the role of the Bird within the story of *Jack and the Beanstalk* over the last two sessions. She would refer to the story as, 'the one with the Giant.'

COMMENTARY 20

Caitlin became more directive, more involved as her role evolved. Her language became clear and understandable, not the inaudible speech of her first three sessions. She appeared relaxed, happy, and bright. The observable changes in her behavior were both physical and cognitive.

Session #10: Jack and the Beanstalk

COMMENTARY 21

It was during the last session that the greatest change was noted. Caitlin's interaction, rapport, affect, and overall attitude had altered drastically from the first few sessions to the last one. She had originally seemed depressed and the therapist could not decipher her speech even after asking her to repeat what she had said. She was distracted as the therapist told the stories, and only minimally able, or interested, to act out a small part.

During the last session, she was interactive, verbal, and smiling. She demonstrated positive emotions and better eye contact. She even seemed excitable. She appeared more relaxed, lying down on the sofa to hear the story, with her head resting on a large stuffed teddy bear. She was very conversational and what she was saying could be understood. Our communication flowed. In fact, she talked so freely, it appeared as though she was procrastinating the termination of the last session.

She stated that her favorite part of the story was 'all of it.' The part to be acted out was to be 'all of it.'

COMMENTARY 22

She was clearly more attentive and focused. Caitlin's involvement had increased greatly over the ten sessions. Her ability to express herself both verbally and symbolically had developed as several levels of therapeutic communication unfolded. She progressed from single-word responses to full and complete sentences. The intonations in her voice were more expressive.

Jack / Therapist:	Little Bird, what am I going to do? Mother wants me to sell Bessie. What am I going to do?
Bird / Caitlin:	You can get things…the harp.
Jack:	The harp?
Bird:	From the giant.
Jack:	What giant?
Bird:	You can get the magic beans.
Jack:	Magic beans? I've never heard of magic beans. What do they do?
Bird:	They're magic.
Jack:	Where do I get them from?
Bird:	The old man.
Jack:	So, you think I should sell Bessie.
Bird:	You can switch.
Jack:	You mean trade? All right, if you say so, I'll do it.
Bird:	OK.

Narrator / Therapist: Well, the boy didn't know what to think, so he took Bessie the cow [*mooo*] over to the market and a man jumped out and said…

Man / Therapist: Hey, you…little boy. Would you like to trade for the cow? I've got some beans!

Jack: Beans for a cow? Wait, let me talk to my friend. Oh, Bird, that man wants me to trade beans for a cow. I don't think it's a good idea, do you?

Bird: Yes.

Jack: Yes? I should do it? For beans?

Bird: [*Nods yes*]

Jack: Why would I want beans?

Bird: They're magic.

Jack: They're magic? Are you sure? I don't want to give up Bessie.

Bird: [*She sings*] You're going to have some money!

Jack: Really, you think I should do it? Sell Bessie for beans… [pause]. All right, I'll do it!

Narrator: After Jack and the Bird tell Mother what they have done, she gets angry and they are sent to their room.

Jack: Little Bird, what do I do now?

Bird: We can go climb up the beanstalk.

Jack: Beanstalk, what are you talking about?

Bird: It's coming.

Jack: A beanstalk? No way, silly Bird, you've been reading way too many stories.

Narrator: Jack didn't even believe the Bird. So Jack went to sleep, into a deep sleep, but the next morning the Bird woke him up.

Jack: [*Gets awakened by the Bird*] What is it? You've gotten me in so much trouble. What? Look at what?

Bird: [*Nudges Jack, and points to beanstalk as projected onto the oxygen tank.*] Look out the window.

Jack: It's a beanstalk! You were right. Should we climb it?

Bird: Yes.

COMMENTARY 23

As the story unfolds, Caitlin's role of the Bird has evolved from the helper to the role of visionary. She now foreshadows and predicts what will be happening. The qualities of the visionary are characterized by a 'prophetic wisdom and insight'. The function of the visionary includes an ability to 'see beyond external events' and to 'predict the future on the basis of such spiritual knowing' (Landy 1993, pp.232–233). The style of this role is presentational due to its innate need for reflection and critical thought.

Through the progression of dramatizations, Caitlin had become the bird of wisdom, knowing what the future held and that everything would turn out for the best. This fiction related to her everyday life in that Caitlin needed to know that there was hope that everything would turn out well for her.

After the ten dramatherapy sessions with Caitlin had been completed, an interview was scheduled with her primary nurse. According to Caitlin's nurse, over the summer months, which were the weeks when her drama-therapy took place, Caitlin's need for oxygen decreased, from one liter to only three-quarters of a liter. For the first time, there was hope that she may be able to go off of the 24-hour oxygen. According to Dr Alistair Martin-Smith, Educational Theatre Specialist:

> The issue of dependence versus independence from oxygen is signifi-cant in Caitlin's case, since she appears to have conceptualized the notion of independence from her dramatization of Jack and the Beanstalk. Since she has been dependent on oxygen since birth, the dramatherapy may have allowed her to physically explore the concept of independence from oxygen, even if only temporarily. (personal communication, September 17 1998)

Caitlin created an original role not found in most of the stories and then developed it as the weeks unfolded. The self-expression and communica-tion, which were exerted by an initially inaudible child, were significant. It was the role of the Bird, which could fly unencumbered and freely up to the heavens to face its greatest fears and to succeed, that allowed Caitlin to succeed in facing her own fears.

Excerpts of a transcription of a selected dramatherapy session, which includes the story of Jack and the Beanstalk as was told, is at the end of this case. CMAS-R test results will be discussed both individually and cu-mulatively in Appendix A.

Discussion

Caitlin demonstrated a marked change in behavior from the first few dramatherapy sessions to the last. She was initially fidgety, inattentive, preoccupied, and distractible. Her affect was flat. Caitlin exhibited poor eye contact and was nearly inaudible. She appeared visibly distressed and under stress. It was initially frustrating for the therapist to try to connect with Caitlin. When she did speak, which was minimally, she couldn't be understood. Even upon asking her to repeat what she had said, her language still could not be comprehended because of the speech impediment.

Her behavior progressed drastically over ten weeks. By the last few sessions, Caitlin was no longer fidgety or distractible. She was focused and motivated. Her affect was bright. She was smiling and laughing for the first time. Her eye contact was steady and everything she said could be understood. Caitlin was no longer listless or seemingly depressed. The therapist and Caitlin could communicate verbally by having lengthy, animated conversations and could communicate through the dramatizations. There were no longer any indications of stress. She looked relaxed. A transformation had taken place.

The Stress Measure, which is an observational tool based on the Symptoms of Stress by psychologist Michael Antoni (Pelletier 1993), indicated a vast improvement in Caitlin's stress level (see Appendix A). The three major sources of stress in chronically ill children have been cited as separation anxiety, loss of control, and fear of bodily harm or death. The stress-related issues that emerged within the dramatizations with Caitlin also suggest a reduction in stress. She began exploring the issue of separation anxiety during the initial sessions. She was actually in the role of the Mother at first, one who may be directly related to separation anxiety. Having acted through this initial issue, Caitlin then, by becoming the Bird, began to delve into the issue of fear of bodily harm or death. This issue became very pronounced in Caitlin's dramatizations, which began with struggles against the Wolf, then the Witch, and finally the biggest threat, the Giant. Fear of bodily harm or death was the most progressive and heightened issue expressed. Through her role-playing, Caitlin was increasingly able to face more fearful issues regarding bodily harm and death. There was an overall sense of fighting to maintain control, as opposed to experiencing a loss of control. The exploration of these pertinent stress-related issues had been expressed through the dramatherapy sessions. Caitlin's ability and motivation to fight her fears reached a crescendo by the last session, as stress was clearly reduced through the dramatizations.

Interviews of parents and staff suggested that Caitlin enjoyed drama and was enthusiastic about attending each session. She displayed a bright and positive affect when she referred to drama. Caitlin's father stated that his daughter responded to the drama sessions 'very favorably.' During a post-interview, he added, 'I think it [the drama] was wonderful. Will she be able to have drama again?' (Mr B, personal communication, October 6 1997). The staff social worker noticed a positive change in Caitlin's behavior since she had the dramatherapy sessions. This change included her ability to 'stay in her seat better' and to 'wait her turn.' These improvements may relate to a decrease in stress. According to her primary care nurse, 'Caitlin's need for oxygen decreased greatly. For the first time there is a possibility she may be able to go off it' (DS, personal communication, September 17 1997). Overall, the interviews suggest that Caitlin not only had a positive experience with drama, but also had some observable change that may indicate a reduction in stress.

The Children's Manifest Anxiety Scale – Revised (CMAS-R) was administered as both a pre- and post-test. For a younger child of Caitlin's age of 6, combined with a language disorder, the test is considered to be somewhat less reliable and less valid. Caitlin's score of 16 remained the same for both tests, indicating no change in stress levels. This also suggests that there was no increase in stress (see Appendix A).

Overall, based on clinical observations, stress measures and the analyzed case study itself, it appears as though Caitlin's stress was reduced through dramatherapy intervention. This, in turn, may have benefited her medical condition, as was indicated by her need for less oxygen.

Six-Month Follow-Up

Caitlin's health had improved during and immediately following the dramatherapy treatment. There was discussion of the possibility of

Caitlin weaning herself off 24-hour-a-day oxygen. Unfortunately, over the following six months her medical condition worsened slightly. She couldn't run or play with other children, and her oxygen had to be increased from three-quarters to one liter. Caitlin had to be hospitalized from December 17 through December 21 1997 because of an infection from her catheter (DS, personal communication, March 23 1998). Caitlin's medical condition is now stable.

Behaviorally, Caitlin is more outgoing and not as shy as before. She is reportedly getting along well with others and has been nominated as class representative. She is referred to as 'happy-go-lucky' with no behavioral indications of stress (DS, personal communication, March 23 1998). Caitlin's health is considered to be the most fragile of any of the subjects of this study because of the nature of her serious illness.

Note

A one-year follow-up found that Caitlin was off oxygen except at night.

Transcript of selected session

Caitlin: Selected Session #9 (9/4/97)

Therapist:	(Speaking into a microphone.) Hello it's Caitlin and Miss Carol here for drama. Would you like to say hello, Caitlin?
Caitlin:	Hello.
Therapist:	We're happy to be back for drama and we'll let you know what story we decide upon. Talk to you soon.
Therapist:	Oh, it's one of those squeezy balls. If you feel like you've got stress or you're upset, you squeeze it and it makes you feel better. Did you really go away for vacation somewhere?
Caitlin:	No. I just went school shopping.
Therapist:	Oh you did? – for back to school?
Caitlin:	Yeah. I needed some stuff.
Therapist:	And you just started school up again didn't you?

Caitlin:	Yeah.
Therapist:	With your teachers back and everyone's back in school. It looks like some new children in the classroom.
Caitlin:	It looks funny.
Therapist:	Ahhh.
Caitlin:	I like my naps. And I like Lassie.
Therapist:	Oh do you? You like Lassie?
Caitlin:	Yeah.
Therapist:	I like Lassie too. I didn't know you liked Lassie. Lassie's my second favorite dog.
Caitlin:	My Mom said – me and my Dad said 'I like the cat and I like the purest of dogs.'
Therapist:	Your Dad likes dogs? Guess what? I have one, I have a dog [*whisper*] and a cat.
Caitlin:	Does the dog chase cats?
Therapist: [*Laugh*]	My dog chases my cat. I feel so bad for the cat. She's got her claws though.
Caitlin:	I have a cat and a dog.
Therapist:	Really both? But it's true, dogs like to chase cats.
Caitlin:	I know because when my Dad and Uncle Mark came and then I was eating it and then the dog took it and he wanted to eat it.
Therapist:	No. The dog wanted to eat it?
Caitlin:	Yeah – eat it.
Therapist:	Oh no. Those dogs are so hungry. If you had a hamburger in your hand a dog would come right over and eat it.
Caitlin:	I know – if he had a big mouth he can eat it.
Therapist:	My dog has a very big mouth. My dog's a very big dog and…
Caitlin:	Is he this big?
Therapist:	Guess how big. He's this tall, he's this big, he probably weighs more than you. How much do you weigh?

Caitlin:	I don't know.
Therapist:	Maybe you weigh 50? 40, 50? Guess how much my dog weighs? 70, 75.
Caitlin:	Does that mean a lot of pounds?
Therapist:	That's a lot of pounds. He's this tall, he's a sheepdog. He's this tall and he's this long and he's so big I can't pick him up. That's how big he is.
Caitlin:	And you can't take him a bath?
Therapist:	When I give him a bath, he gets wet, I get wet, everything gets wet, he shakes and everybody gets sprayed with water. It's a big chore and his hair's long so it takes me hours to comb.
Caitlin:	Does it stay like that?
Therapist:	Well he fluffs up. He looks just like a stuffed animal – when I brush him. He looks just like a stuffed animal. Oh guess what I did? One day I went to McDonald's.
Caitlin:	Yeah.
Therapist:	I bought him a hamburger. I bought it for him. I got him a hamburger and he ate it. He loved it.
Caitlin:	Does he still like hamburgers?
Therapist:	Yes, you know what else? His birthday's this weekend.
Caitlin:	Who's coming to his birthday?
Therapist:	Well, I don't know who to invite – if I should invite some other dogs [*laughter*] and have a dog birthday. He'll be six years old.
Caitlin:	Does that mean he's going to be as big as me?
Therapist:	How old are you?
Caitlin:	Umm…first grade.
Therapist:	How old are you? Are you six? Seven?
Caitlin:	Inh…inh. First grade.
Therapist:	You're in the first grade? Do you like first grade?
Caitlin:	Yeah.
Therapist:	That's such a big thing. Is your teacher nice?

Caitlin:	We get rules in the class.
Therapist:	Oh you get rules?
Caitlin:	Yeah.
Therapist:	Oh. You don't have to worry about those rules here.
Caitlin:	And my class has them.
Therapist:	Well rules are nice for school.
Caitlin:	I don't like rules.
Therapist:	No – me either. [*laughter*]
Caitlin:	Because you can't do anything.
Therapist:	Oh really. Oh no. But the good news is that you'll probably be learning some stuff right?
Caitlin:	Yeah. We get to make tacos.
Therapist:	Are you having tacos today?
Caitlin:	No – we used to make them but not anymore.
Therapist:	Oh, because you had them this summer.
Caitlin:	Yeah.
Therapist:	Heh, did you get new tennis shoes too?
Caitlin:	Yeah, I got them when I went to the beach.
Therapist:	Oh did you?
Caitlin:	Yeah, we have hermit crabs.
Therapist:	You have what?
Caitlin:	[*Louder*] We have hermit crabs.
Therapist:	Hermit crabs?
Caitlin:	They bite Sam. They bite Sam on his arm.
Therapist:	They bit Sam?
Caitlin:	Ah-ha and they bit me when we went home.
Therapist:	Oh no.
Caitlin:	They bit me really hard.
Therapist:	Ouch! Oh that's not fun.
Caitlin:	Allen, his too.

Therapist:	Is Allen your brother?
Caitlin:	Yeah.
Therapist:	Oh, I met your brother one day, he came in to get you. He's your older brother.
Caitlin:	Yeah. His bites a little bit. He's just a little bit.
Therapist:	He took a bite of your brother?
Caitlin:	No – mine did it yesterday – went home. Allen did it too and Allen's bit his arm. It hurt a little bit.
Therapist:	I bet it hurt. I wouldn't want a hermit crab biting me. Not any crab biting me.
Caitlin:	I was playing and it kept biting me.
Therapist:	He must have been hungry. He must have thought you were lunch.
Caitlin:	I know.
Therapist:	All right. Well now let me take a look. We're back for drama. I'm sorry I missed you for two weeks. There's nothing I could do, but now we're back together and I'm going to read you a list of stories – one through five. We have 'til noon today and then you have lunch I think.
Caitlin:	We did all of those stories.
Therapist:	Did we do every one?
Caitlin:	Yes.
Therapist:	Well let me read – *Hansel and Gretel*.
Caitlin:	We did that one.
Therapist:	*Jack and the Beanstalk*.
Caitlin:	We did that one.
Therapist:	*Little Red Riding Hood*.
Caitlin:	We did that one.
Therapist:	*Gingerbread Man*.
Caitlin:	We did that one.
Therapist:	*Three Little Pigs*.

Caitlin:	We did that one.
Therapist:	What are we going to do? We still have to pick one.
Caitlin:	We can do the giant.
Therapist:	Oh – let's do the one with the giant. *Jack and the Beanstalk?*
Caitlin:	Yeah – yeah – yeah.
Therapist:	Now the question is – did I already tell you the story?
Caitlin:	Yes, I want to do it again.
Therapist:	You want me to tell you the story now?
Caitlin:	Yeah, I have that book I think. Yeah, I do, I do.
Therapist:	Do you really?
Caitlin:	Yeah.
Therapist:	All right. I'll tell you the story of *Jack and the Beanstalk* and then we will act out the story.
Caitlin:	OK – we're going to do the same thing.
Therapist:	We are?
Caitlin:	Yeah.
Therapist:	All right then. We'll do the same thing. All right – ready?
Caitlin:	Yep.
Therapist:	Here we go.
Narrator/Therapist:	Once a long time ago and very far away there lived a little boy named Jack and Jack lived with his Mother.
Mother/Therapist:	And one day Mother said, 'Jack! Jack! Come over here!' So Jack came over and Mother said, 'Now, what I'd like you to do is take Bessie down to the market and you sell her and make as much money as you can!'
Jack/Therapist:	And Jack said, 'Mother, I can't sell Bessie. She's our cow. She's our pet and I won't do it!'
Mother:	And Mother said, 'Yes, you will. You will take Bessie. You will sell Bessie because we have no food and no money and it's all we have left to do.'

Cow / Therapist:	So then Jack reluctantly took Bessie the cow and the cow went 'Moooooo' and Jack and Bessie walked along the way.
Man:	And then all of sudden out came this man and the man said, 'Hey little boy, would you like to sell your cow? I'll give you something nice for it.'
Jack:	'Well yes, I'm selling my cow as a matter of fact because my Mother and I have no money. So I would like some money for my cow. How much have you got?'
Man:	'I've got something better than money! I've got beans!'
Jack:	'Beans???'
Man:	'Magic beans!!!' [*With a sly laugh.*]
Jack:	'Magic beans, gee. Magic. Yeah, I'll do it.' So Jack took the magic beans from the man and Jack ran home and said 'Mother, Mother, I did it, I traded the cow!!'
Mother:	'Oh thank heaven. How much did you get? Show me the money. How much did you get? How much money did you get?'
Jack:	'No Mom, not money. I got beans – magic beans.'
Mother:	'Beans??? Beans!!!! That's enough. Go to your room. No dinner. That's the last straw!' She was very, very mad.
Therapist / Narrator:	So Jack went to bed and while he was sleeping up grew a huge beautiful beanstalk.
Jack:	When Jack woke up he looked over and said, 'Ahhh, a beanstalk, I think I'll climb it!'
Narrator:	So Jack began to climb and climb the beanstalk and when he got to the top he looked over and saw a castle.
Woman:	Well, he walked over to the castle, creaked open the door [*creak*] and there was a woman who said, 'What are you doing here in the Giant's castle? Go before he wakes up and sees you. Go or we'll have you for dinner.'
Giant:	And little Jack snuck in and ran behind the chair where the Giant sat and the Giant said, 'Fe, fi, fo, fum, I smell the blood of an Englishman.'

Wife:	And the wife said, 'Oh, dear, you're imagining things. Now then what can I get for you?'
Giant:	'Humph! I'd like my hen!' So the woman went and got the hen and the Giant took the hen and said, 'Lay me an egg, hen!! Lay me an egg!!'
Hen:	And the hen went 'pock-pock-pock-pock' and out came a golden egg.
Giant:	And the Giant said, 'Ha ha ha ha, lay me another egg, hen!!'
Hen:	And the hen laid another egg, 'Pock-pock-pock- pock,' and there was another golden egg.
Giant:	Then the Giant began to get sleepy and fell into a sleep 'Snore…'
Hen:	While he was sleeping Jack got up, ran over and grabbed the golden egg, 'pock-pock-pock-pock.'
Jack:	He ran to the beanstalk and went all the way down the beanstalk and ran over to Mother and said to Mother, 'Mother, Mother, look, a hen! Look, Mother, a hen!'
Mother:	And Mother said, 'Jack where did you get that hen? You didn't steal it did you?'
Jack:	Mother, no, it's from the castle. The hen lays golden eggs, look! Lay me an egg, hen.
Hen:	Pock-pock-pock.
Mother:	And Mother looked and there was a golden egg. 'Ahhh – Jack, this means we'll never be poor again. Oh, Jack, how wonderful!' Then Jack was gone and Mother said, 'Come baaack.'
Giant:	Jack went up the beanstalk and over to the castle, snuck in, sat behind the Giant and the Giant said, 'Wife, bring me my money now!!!' And the wife brought the money and the Giant started to count his gold coins, 'One, two, three, four. Oh, I'm tired, where's my lunch?' And then the Giant fell asleep [*snore*] and little Jack ran out, grabbed the money and ran to the beanstalk.

Mother:	Then all the way down the beanstalk, ran home and gave all the money to Mother who said, 'Jack, where did you get this money? We'll be so rich. Oh Jack, Jack, wait, come back – don't go up…come back…'
Giant:	And Jack for the third and last time went all the way up the beanstalk, over to the castle, snuck in, hid behind the Giant and the Giant said, 'Wife, bring me my harp!' So the wife got the harp and the harp began to sing and the Giant said, 'Sing, harp, sing!'
Harp:	And the harp went, 'Ahhhh-ahhhh-ahhhh-ahhhh.'
Giant:	And the Giant said, 'Sing!!'
Harp:	And the harp went, 'Ahhhh-ahhhh-ahhhh-ahhhh' and the Giant fell into a deep sleep with the beautiful, beautiful music and Jack came out and grabbed the harp. And the harp said, 'Help me master, help me, master, heeeeeeeelp!'
Giant:	And the Giant woke up and said, 'Fe, fi, fo, fum – I smell blood of an Englishman!' And he went out after Jack and Jack ran as fast as he could to the beanstalk – grabbing onto the harp and ran all the way down the beanstalk.
Jack:	'Mother, Mother, quick! Take the harp! Give me an ax!' So he went, grabbed the ax, came over to the beanstalk and chopped! and chopped! and chopped! at the beanstalk. And the Giant fell and was no more. And Jack and his Mother and the hen, and the harp, and the gold lived very, very happily ever after.
Therapist:	And that's the story of Jack and the beanstalk! Now, if you could be anybody in the story, who would you like to be?
Caitlin:	We didn't find the head of this.
Therapist:	It's in the bag somewhere. I'm not sure where. I do have to fix it, I haven't fixed it yet.
Caitlin:	Now where's that Bird? Are you looking for the Bird? I'm sure that it's in there.
Therapist:	Is that who you're going to be today?

Caitlin:	Yeah.
Therapist:	And what does the Bird do?
Caitlin:	[*Is looking in bag.*]
Therapist:	Do you see it?
Caitlin:	Yeah. I saw it.
Therapist:	Good. I'm glad it's there. Now, what part of the story should we do. The whole story or part of the story?
Caitlin:	The whole story.
Therapist:	OK, and who's the Bird going to help.
Caitlin:	The boy.
Therapist:	The little boy. OK, does the little boy have to ask for help or does the Bird just help?
Caitlin:	The Bird will help.
Therapist:	OK, so let's do that and every time the boy needs help, the Bird will help him. Is that how it works? OK. Ready?
Caitlin:	Yeah.
Therapist:	OK, here we go.
Narrator/Therapist:	This is a story called Jack and the Beanstalk. A long time ago and very far away there lived a little boy named Jack.
Mother:	And one day Mother said, 'Jack! Jack, come here! Now you listen to me! I want you to take that cow and take the cow to the marketplace! You've got to sell the cow and make as much money as you can!'
Jack:	And Jack said, 'No. No. I don't want to do it. I'm not going to sell the cow, that's my pet, that's Bessie. We've had her for years Mother.'
Mother:	You've got to do it. We've got no money. You're going to have to do it, Jack.
Jack:	So Jack said to the Bird, 'Mother wants me to sell Bessie. I don't want to do it. What am I going to do?'
The Bird/Caitlin:	The harp.

Jack / Therapist:	The harp?
The Bird / Caitlin:	From the Giant.
Jack / Therapist:	What Giant?
The Bird / Caitlin:	Or the magic beans.
Jack / Therapist:	Magic beans? I've never heard of magic beans. What do they do?
The Bird / Caitlin:	They're magic.
Jack / Therapist:	Magic? Where am I going to get them from?
The Bird / Caitlin:	From the man.
Jack / Therapist:	So you think I should sell Bessie? All right, if you say so.
Caitlin:	You can switch.
Jack / Narrator / Therapist:	Oh, trade? So Jack took the cow, Bessie [*mooooo*], and they went along their merry way and all of a sudden saw a man and the man said, 'Hey, Jack! Little boy. I'll make you a trade for that nice cow. I've got magic beans.' Magic beans, that's what the Bird had told me, something about magic beans but… Bird – should I do it? Trade for magic beans?
The Bird / Caitlin:	How about if you can still keep the cow?
Jack / Therapist:	I can still keep the cow?
The Bird / Caitlin:	Yeah.
Jack / Therapist:	Because I can't part with my pet.
The Bird / Caitlin:	Yes.
Jack / Therapist:	All right. I'm going to take the beans, but you can't have my cow. Maybe some other day I'll repay you.
Jack:	So Jack took the beans and the cow and went back home and said, 'Mother! Mother! Look!'
Mother:	What are you doing with Bessie? Didn't you get any money for her?
Jack:	No, Mother, I got beans…beans…magical beans.
Mother:	Beans? Magic beans? Go to your room.
Jack:	But I…

Mother:	No buts.
Jack:	But I... [*something drops on the floor*]
Mother:	Go!
Narrator/Therapist:	So poor Jack went to his room and went to sleep for the night. The Bird woke Jack up the next day – actually the Bird woke him up – he was sleeping [*snores*].
Jack:	Ummh – go away! [*More snores*] What? What? Who is it? Huhhh...it's a Bird. Who is it?
Narrator:	Look at what?
Caitlin:	Out the window.
Narrator:	Huhhh [*with surprise*]...what's that?
Caitlin:	A beanstalk.
Narrator:	From the beans? The magic beans made it? [*Whispering*] Do you think I should climb it? Do you think I should go up and see what's at the top?
Caitlin:	I guess so.
Narrator:	Do you want to go with me?
Caitlin:	Yeah.
Narrator:	OK, come on, let's go!! So now Jack and the Bird went over to the beanstalk and they climbed and the Bird flew all the way up.
Jack:	Look! It's a castle.
Narrator:	Should we go in? Come on, let's go! So the Bird and the little boy went in and hid behind the Giant's chair.
Giant:	And the Giant said, 'Fe, fi, fo, fum. I smell the blood of an Englishman – and a bird.'
Wife:	And the wife said, 'Oh dear, you're imagining things. Here – here – take your hen.'
Giant:	'Lay me a golden egg! [*pock-pock-pock-pock*] Beautiful. Lay me another golden egg. [*pock-pock-pock-pock*] Beautiful. Wife, bring me my lunch!' [*Yawn*] And the giant fell into a deep, deep sleep.

Jack:	While the giant was sleeping – out came the Bird and out came little Jack and Jack said, 'Let's take the hen!! You want him? You hold the eggs. I'll hold the hen. Ready?' So the Bird took the eggs and the boy took the hen and they ran from the beanstalk. 'Let's go!' [*running footsteps*] 'Mother, Mother, look! We got the eggs! We got the hen!'
Mother:	And Mother said, 'We're rich! We're rich! Don't go back up there, Jack.'
Jack:	'Come on, Bird, let's go back.' So they went back to the beanstalk, back into the castle, back behind the chair.
Giant:	And the Giant said, 'Fe, fi, fo, fum. Do I smell a boy and a bird?'
Wife:	And the wife said, 'Oh, dear, you're imagining things.'
Giant:	'What's that I see?'
Wife:	'Dear – just count your money!'
Giant:	'All right. One, two, three, four, what comes after four?' [*sighed*] and then he fell asleep.
Jack:	And then Jack said, 'Come on, let's get the money! I'm going to carry all the money. You can carry in your beak. Quick, let's go to the beanstalk!'
Narrator:	And they went down, down, down the beanstalk as fast as they could [*down, down, down*] and then they ran to Mother.
Jack:	And said, 'Mother, look! The Bird and I got some coins. Look! We'll be rich, rich, rich.'
Mother:	'Jack, I don't want you going back up that beanstalk.'
Jack:	'See you later, Mom.' [*Running footsteps*]
Narrator:	And they went all the way up the beanstalk again and they got to the top and the Giant was sleeping.
Giant:	And the Giant said [*yawning*], 'Bring me my harp. What's that I smell?'
Wife:	Oh, dear, it's nothing, it's just your lunch. Now go ahead and listen to your harp.

Giant:	Play, harp, play.
Harp:	And the harp said, 'Ah-ah-ah-ah-ah-ah.'
Narrator:	And they fell asleep [*snore*] – a deep sleep [*snore*].
Jack:	Come on quick, let's get the harp.
Harp:	But the harp woke up and said, 'Master, heeeeelllllllp!'
Jack and the Harp:	And Jack and the harp went down the beanstalk and said, 'Mother, Mother, give me the ax! Quickly, help me, let's chop the tree! They're coming!'
Narrator:	They got the ax, they went over to the beanstalk and they began to chop, 'Chop, chop, chop.' And down went the beanstalk [*crashing sound*] and the giant was no more. And that's the story of Jack and the beanstalk.

Caitlin and Therapist: [*Clapping*]

Therapist:	Oh good, we've got five minutes left. You know what I want to do?
Caitlin:	When it gets up to there it'll be time?
Therapist:	When it gets on the 12.
Caitlin:	That's 12?
Therapist:	When the big hand gets on the 12.
Caitlin:	Right there.
Therapist:	Yeah. The big black hand.
Caitlin:	That right there.
Therapist:	Yeah – the one that's near the 11.
Caitlin:	Right there with the 0 and the 1?
Therapist:	The long black hand. When it touches 12 the 1 and the 2.
Caitlin:	Right there the 1 and the 2?
Therapist:	Yes. We're almost done. But you know what, before we go today I want to give you this little questionnaire before I forget. It's a yes and no thing, remember? We'll still have Drama again.
Caitlin:	OK.

Therapist:	Hah? I'm going to give this to you so we don't have to worry about it. OK, ready? Just say yes or no. I have trouble making up my mind. Yes or no.
Caitlin:	No.
Therapist:	I get nervous when things do not go the right way for me.
Caitlin:	Yes.
Therapist:	Others seem to do things easier than I can.
Caitlin:	Yes.
Therapist:	I like everyone I know.
Caitlin:	Yes.
Therapist:	I have trouble getting my breath.
Caitlin:	No.
Therapist:	I worry a lot of the time.
Caitlin:	Yes/No.
Therapist:	I am afraid of a lot of things.
Caitlin:	Yes.
Therapist:	I am always kind.
Caitlin:	Yes.
Therapist:	I get mad easily.
Caitlin:	Yes.
Therapist:	I worry about what my parents will say to me.
Caitlin:	Yes.
Therapist:	I feel that others do not like the way I do things.
Caitlin:	Yes.
Therapist:	I always have good manners.
Caitlin:	Yes.
Therapist:	It's hard for me to get to sleep at night.
Caitlin:	No.
Therapist:	I worry about what other people think about me.

Caitlin:	No.
Therapist:	I feel alone even when there are people with me.
Caitlin:	Yes.
Therapist:	I am always good.
Caitlin:	Yes.
Therapist:	Often I feel sick in my stomach.
Caitlin:	Yes.
Therapist:	My feelings get hurt easily.
Caitlin:	No.
Therapist:	My hands feel sweaty.
Caitlin:	Yes.
Therapist:	I am always nice to everyone.
Caitlin:	Yeah/No.
Therapist:	I am tired a lot.
Caitlin:	Yes.
Therapist:	I worry about what is going to happen.
Caitlin:	No.
Therapist:	Other children are happier than I.
Caitlin:	Yes.
Therapist:	I tell the truth every single time.
Caitlin:	Yes.
Therapist:	I have bad dreams.
Caitlin:	No.
Therapist:	My feelings get hurt easily when I am fussed at.
Caitlin:	No.
Therapist:	I feel someone will tell me I do things the wrong way.
Caitlin:	No.
Therapist:	I never get angry.
Caitlin:	Yes.
Therapist:	I wake up scared some of the time.

Caitlin: Yes.

Therapist: I worry when I go to bed at night.

Caitlin: Yes, I mean no.

Therapist: It's hard for me to keep my mind on my schoolwork.

Caitlin: Yes.

Therapist: I never say things I shouldn't.

Caitlin: No, I mean yes.

Therapist: I wiggle in my seat a lot.

Caitlin: Yes.

Therapist: I am nervous.

Caitlin: Yes.

Therapist: A lot of people are against me.

Caitlin: Yes.

Therapist: I never lie.

Caitlin: Yes.

Therapist: I often worry about something bad happening to me.

Caitlin: No.

Therapist: All right – we're done. I wanted to finish our test. We'll have more Drama time. But let me put the date. But anyway I wanted to tell you – your story was very good when you were the Bird. You did such a nice job today. Should we say goodbye?

Caitlin: Yes.

Therapist: Goodbye until next time.

Caitlin: Bye.

Therapist: Can you tell everybody who you were today?

Caitlin: The Bird.

Therapist: And what did the Bird do?

Caitlin: He helped the boy.

Therapist: And was the Bird a big help?

Caitlin: Yes.

Therapist:	I would like to say the Bird was a very big help and I don't think Jack could have done it without that Bird.
Caitlin:	He did.
Therapist:	Goodbye for now.
Caitlin:	Bye.
Therapist:	We'll see you next week.

lavender and cornerless, the moon rattles like a fragment of angry candy

E.E. Cummings

The Angel Wolf

This second case further validates the work, by the recurring themes and patterns that emerge throughout the stories, which relate to Tasha's illness. This seemingly introverted and soft-spoken child was able to explore serious issues, including death, through her role-playing.

Background

Tasha is a seven-and-a-half-year-old girl, diagnosed with IDDM (Insulin Dependent Diabetes Mellitus). She was first diagnosed during the spring of 1996. She was then hospitalized for two months and had difficulty with stabilization. Tasha presently receives injections of insulin twice daily, before breakfast and before dinner. These injections are administered by a registered nurse. She must also use an Accu-Check instrument, which is a self-administered 'needle-stick' in the finger, four to five times daily to monitor her blood glucose levels. All of these procedures are invasive and painful. Tasha is on a strict diet outlined by the American Diabetes Association (ADA) which includes 1800 calories per day, no candy or sugars, and few carbohydrates. Tasha's complete diagnoses are as follows:

Axis I: Attention Deficit Hyperactivity Disorder (Inattentive Type)

Axis II: Borderline Intellectual Functioning

Axis III: IDDM.

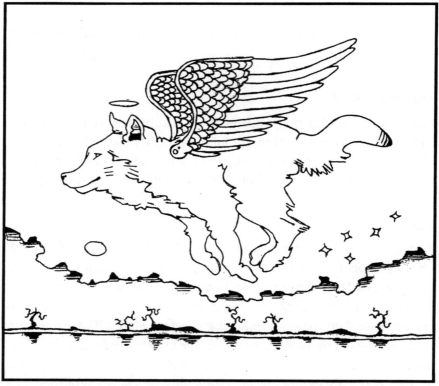

Figure 4.3 'Then the Wolf came back to life, and he was an Angel then' (illustration by Laurence Muleh 2001)

In addition to juvenile diabetes, Tasha is considered to be below average to borderline in her cognitive, academic, and memory skills. According to her medical chart, she has poor comprehension skills and is inattentive and impulsive. She is considered to be withdrawn, anxious, and depressed at home. Tasha needed to repeat the first grade.

Tasha has mild expressive and receptive delay in language. She is considered cooperative at the school/partial day hospital program and denies physical complaints. She is described as shy and quiet and does not engage in conversation often. Tasha can't eat breakfast with the other children whenever her blood sugar is too high. She must sit and wait for a half an hour after her injection, while watching the other children eat. She doesn't complain. According to the social worker's notes, Tasha is not 'tuned in,' but in a 'daze.' She has difficulty with too many stimuli. Tasha can't remember her sugar count, even when she has just finished testing. It is noted that she would not role-play during group therapy with the social worker.

Tasha's condition is serious and could deteriorate. Her illness is chronic and must be stabilized by her restrictive diet. Childhood diabetes can lead to severe complications including renal failure. Tasha's illness may progress if she does not take care of herself. In addition, she must be strictly monitored. Stress, say Kovacs and Iyengar (1989), is a factor in that it can increase her blood sugar:

> Children with a chronic illness, such as Insulin Dependent Diabetes Mellitus (IDDM), are assumed to be at risk for psychological problems because of the sequence of stresses to which they are exposed. The illness-related stresses include the demands of daily management (e.g. insulin injections, blood glucose monitoring, dietary restrictions), the concomitant constraints on everyday life and one's sense of freedom, the symptoms of the illness itself, as well as hospitalizations and medical complications. (Kovacs and Iyengar 1989, p.620)

Description and Analysis

Session #1: Introduction

Tasha, age seven and a half, initially presented herself as a shy and quiet, yet alert, girl. She appeared cooperative but spoke little. She listened attentively as the therapist talked during their first session. The therapist explained what the drama sessions would entail. Even though the first session was designed as an introduction, with the administration of the pre-test (CMAS-R) and the signing of the assent form, Tasha discovered some assorted puppets belonging to the psychology staff, not part of the pre-selected drama materials for the study. Tasha proceeded to enact a simple role-play, with herself as both doctor and nurse troll puppets, while the therapist was to be the chef troll. The therapist noticed how animated and verbal she became while role-playing with the puppets.

COMMENTARY 1

Tasha had initiated this puppet play, whereas the therapist had no intention of beginning the drama until the next session. The use of puppets is more distant and therefore safer than other projective techniques such as masks or make-up. This appears to be a safe place for Tasha to start, as she readily and somewhat prematurely begins. During this brief interchange with the therapist in the role of chef, the issue of Tasha's own restrictive diet emerged. The chef is the role whose function is to cook and prepare food.

She assumed the role of the medical staff, and told the chef that 'you're OK' and 'not sick' after taking the chef's temperature. Then Tasha took a lion puppet and tried to eat the therapist's giraffe puppet. She petted the giraffe puppet. Next, the lion puppet (Tasha) began to eat all of the other puppets. She invites the therapist to join her and together they consumed the puppet menagerie. She explained that they wouldn't eat the doctor puppet, then quickly said that they would, even though they shouldn't. Every puppet was devoured by the growling lion.

COMMENTARY 2

Tasha's aggression in the role of the lion, and her uncontrollable oral fixation, was indicative of her illness and the restrictive diet to which she must adhere so strictly. She cannot eat what she wants like the other children. Tasha's ambivalence towards doctors was also expressed by this initial role playing. It was clear how much she had to express. She initiated this puppet play completely on her own, with no encouragement or request from the therapist.

Session #2: Little Red Riding Hood

During the first actual dramatherapy session with Tasha, she chose what was to be her preferred and most selected story, *Little Red Riding Hood*. She chose to play the role of Little Red Riding Hood after listening intently as the therapist told her the story.

COMMENTARY 3

The story of Little Red Riding Hood *proved to be a comfortable tale for Tasha. 'The story is the container of one's roles... a role can exist without a story, but requires a story in order to communicate its essence' (Landy 1993, p.31). The familiarity of this story would provide a way for Tasha to begin to invoke and explore roles. The essence of these roles will come to fruition as the sessions unfold.*

Although she appeared shy and somewhat withdrawn, the therapist noticed that Tasha made very good eye contact and possessed a positive affect. Despite her diagnoses that include Attention Deficit and Hyperactivity Disorder, she was able to sit and listen to the story from beginning to end, with appropriate expression.

After the story was told, Tasha explored the contents of the drama bag and selected a white furry bunny mask to wear as Little Red. She also wrapped a large scarf around her shoulders to be the red cape of Red Riding Hood. She directed the therapist to be the Wolf by using a wolf puppet. She found a plastic case to be the basket of goodies. She also requested that the therapist be the Mom in the first scene. She played the role simply, yet according to the story. Tasha was minimally verbal, even in the role. The infamous scene unfolded according to the story.

Little Red / Tasha:	Grandmother, what big ears you have.
Wolf / Therapist:	[*Pretends to be granny*] The better to hear you with, my dear!
Little Red:	Grandmother, what big eyes you have!
Wolf:	The better to see you with, my dear!

Little Red: Grandmother, what big teeth you have!

Wolf: The better to gobble you up. [*Wolf lunges and gobbles up Little Red.*]

COMMENTARY 4

When the Wolf gobbled Little Red, Tasha actually cringed and flinched. This moment of fear may have been cathartic for Tasha. It is this moment of recognition in combination with the expression of fear that appeared to have an unconscious effect on Tasha. This also suggests the issue of fear of bodily harm or death. After Little Red is devoured, she literally hides under a cloth to pretend she was gobbled up. Not only is Little Red harmed, with death seemingly imminent, but she has also been eaten whole by the Wolf. The Wolf consumes Little Red. A pattern of devouring is emerging within this young diabetic's role-playing.

The Wolf represents disorder and lack of harmony with his overpowering motivations, that of greed and guile (Rowland 1973). It is the Wolf's own appetite that seals his fate. This relates to the impending threat of the diabetic child's own appetite. The Wolf's appetite is all-consuming, even insatiable. During Little Red Riding Hood, *the Wolf eats two people. It is during this notorious scene that the physical senses are unleashed from ears to eyes to mouth. These senses are all active when eating. According to Heuscher (1994), author of* A Psychiatric Study of Myths and Fairy Tales, *all of the hearing, seeing, touching and tasting create an environment of sensory sensations.*

Little Red Riding Hood *is a story of temptation, not unlike Tasha's daily struggle with temptation. Tasha's temptations are mandated by a restrictive diet. In addition, Little Red Riding Hood's own cloak is red, the color of blood, which is not only a perceived root of Tasha's illness, but is also what she has to observe four or five times a day with her Accu-Check needle. Yet, during this first dramatherapy session, Tasha finds some distance through the role of the protagonist and will continue in the role of the protagonist for many sessions to come.*

As the first story ended, the Huntsman (therapist) saved Little Red (Tasha) and the Grandmother. This is in accordance with the fairy tale (Grimm 1812). Tasha removed the white bunny mask and helped to return the drama materials.

COMMENTARY 5

Tasha seemed proud of her accomplishments and her ability to escape temptation. The white, furry bunny mask accentuated the character of Little Red Riding Hood, and created an original role. The innocence, frailty, and naivety of a bunny seemed to complement those same characteristics of Little Red. Little Red Riding Hood is universally loved because of these trusting characteristics which actually lead her to temporary demise. There is something about the big bad Wolf that is likable or he holds no power over us (Bornstein 1988). The mask gives Tasha some distance and the furry white bunny itself is comforting for her. This bunny/Little Red duality seems to be a safe place for Tasha to be in, especially to start in her exploration of self through role-playing.

Session #3: Hansel and Gretel

During the third session, Tasha entered willingly. She appeared shy, quiet, and actually sweet in nature. Her eyes were big and bright. Tasha appeared eager for her drama session. When asked, she immediately recalled the story of *Little Red Riding Hood* from last week.

COMMENTARY 6

This is a child who was described, by more than one staff member, as having a short-term memory problem. Apparently, she is not able to remember her Accu-Check reading moments after she is given the information. Yet, her first dramatherapy story is very memorable for her. It appears as though she may be able to remember if she so desires. If it's something positive, or of interest to her, then she can remember quite vividly.

There is a relationship between drama and memory as suggested by specialists in the field. People learn by doing. According to Creative Arts Therapist Mary Anne Bartley: 'We remember 20 per cent of what we hear; 40 per cent of what we hear and see, but 75 per cent of what we see, hear, and do' (1997, pp.36–39). Since we learn through memory, this may suggest a relationship between memory and drama.

She listened to the choices of fairy tales and the therapist asked her to choose one. She selected the story of *Hansel and Gretel*. After listening attentively to the story, she selected the role of Gretel. She selected a black, furry cat mask and a gold crown to wear. Then she selected the white, furry bunny mask and a silver-sparkled top hat to wear as Hansel.

She was to play both protagonists. Tasha gave the therapist a witch hat to wear as the Witch.

COMMENTARY 7

Again, she is using furry, comforting animal masks to further protect the protagonist(s) of the story. The use of masks is less distant than the puppets that Tasha used during the first session, because they are worn on the face. Yet, Tasha's use of animal masks to portray the roles of Hansel and Gretel suggests an element of safety. She also decided to play both the part of the brother Hansel and the sister Gretel. It seems there is more safety for Tasha in playing the dual roles. She is better able to identify with the hero, by becoming both protagonists. It is a stronger connection. The child's identification with the protagonists can result in a catharsis because of this very connection. Tasha was strengthening her identification with the protagonist by becoming both heroes. Role-playing both protagonists at once also suggests a need for control. Tasha experienced some feelings of a loss of control manifested by her illness.

Tasha stated her favorite part of the story was 'the whole story.' She said she wanted to act out the story 'from the start.' Yet, as she began her drama, she actually started as Hansel and Gretel discovered the gingerbread house.

Gretel/Tasha:	Look, there is a gingerbread house!
Narrator/Therapist:	Suddenly, Gretel spotted a beautiful gingerbread house. It was like nothing she had ever seen. She and Hansel decided to try it.
Gretel:	[*Begins to eat*] Mmmm.
Narrator:	The house tasted so good! It was made of wonderful gingerbread, gumdrops, candy canes, licorice, and icing. Hansel and Gretel ate and ate.

COMMENTARY 8

As the therapist watched, Tasha ate the imaginary candy house with lusty fervor. An insulin-dependent child was given the opportunity to devour any child's dream treat. For Tasha, unable to eat sweets, the moment in the dramatization was cathartic. She's clearly unable to eat sweets because of her illness, yet was able to eat an entire candy house through the drama. In

*the role of the narrator, the therapist paused to see if she would continue to
eat. As the narrator, the therapist must be aware of the patient's needs so that
the pace of the story can be manipulated accordingly. It was important for
Tasha to devour the candy house without limits, so the narrator improvised
in order to allow for this necessary exploration. The therapist didn't want
to encourage her to eat through the narration, unless she was motivated to
do so for herself. She continued to eat.*

Narrator: [*Pause, as Hansel and Gretel continue to eat.*] The house was
delicious! Just imagine sugarplums, lemondrops, pepper-
mint swirls and lollipop trim.

Gretel: Mmm. Hansel, try this. [*Continues to eat the imaginary house
with much passion. She didn't stop.*]

COMMENTARY 9

*Tasha continued eating the house in a relentless fashion. The therapist
noticed an unfolding pattern of devouring, which was expressed through
previous stories. Tasha's oral fixation became clearer with each session.
The temptation of a candy house is great for any child, yet for Tasha this
fantasy proved to be a very powerful reality. Her daily temptation became
restrained. According to Tasha's primary nurse, 'Although she adheres to
her diet here at the hospital, she gives her mom a hard time at home. She's
used to getting what she wants.' The social worker confirmed this:*

> *...I know that at home she cries when she's not supposed to have
> something, and she cries until her mother gives in to her, and then she'll
> eat things that she's not supposed to. She doesn't do that here, she's
> pretty good. But how do you expect a 6- to 7-year-old to accept that
> she's not supposed to eat what other people can eat. That's pretty hard.*
> *(JM, personal communications, September 21 1997)*

*It is this delectable gingerbread house that lures the children to their deaths
(Thomas 1989). For Tasha, this is actually the case. She will never be able
to eat a gingerbread house, or even a slice of gingerbread, because it would
lead to serious complications. When Tasha, in the role of Gretel, says,
'Hansel, try this,' she is actually giving herself permission to consume
forbidden sweets, since she is in the role of Hansel too.*

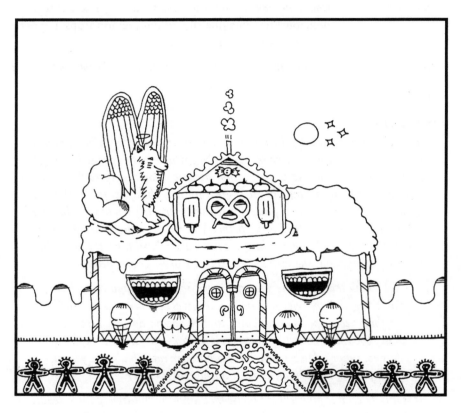

Figure 4.4 The sweet scent of the candy house filled the air…it was every child's dream treat (illustration by Laurence Muleh 2001)

Session #4: Little Red Riding Hood

During the fourth session, Tasha selected *Little Red Riding Hood* once again. She chose the character of Little Red Riding Hood, and refers to her as the 'little girl.'

COMMENTARY 10

> *Tasha was more verbal and animated than before. She seemed eager to participate and appeared less inhibited. Her initial shyness quickly dissolved as her innate desire to express herself through dramatic play manifested itself.*

Therapist:	You can use anything in the bag or any make-up to do...
Tasha:	[*Interjects*] Make-up.
Therapist:	...the story. You want to use make-up for the little girl?
Tasha:	Yeah.
Therapist:	OK.
Tasha:	[*Takes out bird puppet.*] This could be the bird that ate all the crumbs.
Therapist:	Yes, exactly. The bird that ate all the crumbs.
Tasha:	Yeahee, the bread crumbs?

COMMENTARY 11

> *Although we were planning to act out the story of* Little Red Riding Hood, *she was referring to a scene from* Hansel and Gretel. *Another incident involving one's eating leading to potential harm. The Bird eats all the bread crumbs and the children are then completely lost, with no way home.*

Therapist:	Shall we look in the make-up bag?
Tasha:	Yeah [*pause*] where is it?
Therapist:	It's right here.
Tasha:	I saw it.
Therapist:	OK. Here we go.

The therapist explained that the make-up must be removed five minutes before the session was over and Tasha agreed. Tasha was shown the various types of make-up that were available for her use. There were make-up pencils, crayons, foundations, and liquids, all in various colors. There was also 'sparkle' make-up.

Therapist:	OK. We're going to do the story of *Little Red Riding Hood* and you're going to be the 'little girl.' What color do you want to use first? For make-up for the little girl's face?
Tasha:	Uhh...red.
Therapist:	Do you want red for cheeks?
Tasha:	No.
Therapist:	Do you want lips?
Tasha:	No, heart.

The therapist gave Tasha a choice whether she wanted to apply the make-up herself or wanted the therapist to do it. At first she said she would do it, so she was warned not to put any make-up too close to her eyes. Upon hearing this warning she changed her mind and asked the therapist to apply the make-up for that session.

COMMENTARY 12

Tasha's request for the therapist to apply the make-up was apparently due to the warning. This relates to the issue of fear of bodily harm. Tasha was more secure in allowing the therapist to apply her make-up, according to Tasha's specifications.

The therapist assumed that Tasha would make her face look like a 'little girl's.' However, she chose specific symbols and selected colors to be drawn onto her face like a picture. The therapist must always go where the child needs to go, and be careful not to assume anything. At her request, the therapist proceeded to draw a red heart, first on one cheek, then on the other. Then she asked for 'lips.' She selected black for her lips.

COMMENTARY 13

As Tasha's lips blackened, the therapist noticed the contrast between her lips and the bright red hearts placed symmetrically on her cheeks. She had blackened her mouth, the focal point of her oral restrictions, and contrasted this with the symbol for the heart, which is an integral part of her blood disease. She then asked for some stars. She chose white for the stars. The researcher noted the contrast of the white, black, and red make-up, as related by Thomas (1989):

> *White, black, and red are favored over all other colors. The triad's universal popularity lies in the stark contrast the colors pose to each other. White and black exemplify and symbolize all contrasts perceived in the natural and supernatural worlds: day and night, the known and the hidden, life and death. Red represents blood. Together white, black and red are the most emotional and have the most symbolic content of any color groupings. (Thomas 1989, p.126)*

Tasha proceeded to act out the role of 'the little girl.'

COMMENTARY 14

The symbolic make-up added a new dimension to her dramatizations. Tasha seemed more confident in role-playing with the specifically designed make-up she wore. Tasha was to use make-up as a projective technique for several sessions to come. It was as though Tasha was using the counter-colors of white and black to symbolize a balance, yet it was the blood red that upset the equilibrium. Black and white are opposite colors as they represent all or nothing in the color spectrum. This may have been reflective of Tasha's oral struggle with the recurring pattern of restriction and abundance of food. The blood red color may have been reflective of her disease although the significance of the color choices is conjecture. Landy (1994) discusses make-up:

> *Make-up is an alternative form of masking. It tends to be less distanced than mask work, as it is applied directly onto the face and cannot be separated from the face itself. Like the mask, make-up has its roots in shamanistic, magical practices. (Landy 1994, pp.145–146)*

Tasha's progression from her initial use of puppets, to masks to make-up indicates a decrease in her need for distance. This pattern suggests that she may be feeling more able to express herself with less distance. Tasha was becoming less inhibited and more comfortable in her role-playing as indicated by this transition. She literally had let go of the masks from earlier sessions, and was to express herself, symbolically, through the use of make-up.

Session #5: Hansel and Gretel

During the fifth session, an aura of ease spread over Tasha. She seemed very comfortable, and was much more verbal than before. She was conversational and animated, forming complete sentences rather than single-word responses. At first she selected the story of *Little Red Riding Hood*, but then changed her mind and instead selected *Hansel and Gretel*. As in a previous session, she chose the characters of both Hansel and Gretel. Rather than masks, she wanted to use make-up and asked the therapist to apply it for her. She started with black and asked for a black heart. She proceeded to request a red heart for the other cheek. Again, she wanted white stars. This time she added some yellow stripes.

COMMENTARY 15

A transformation occurred as Tasha painstakingly selected each color and each specific symbol to be applied to her face. The process of applying the make-up was carefully orchestrated. Tasha observed the transformation in a mirror as it unfolded on her face. 'In dramatherapy, make-up, like mask work, is a projective device that conceals in order to reveal parts of the self not yet fully expressed in everyday life' (Landy 1994, p.146). She actually watched in the mirror as the specifically requested designs were applied. She reminded the therapist that she said she was going to bring in Q-tips and more cold cream, which she did say, and did forget. This doesn't seem to be indicative of a memory loss on her part as was suggested in her medical chart and during her interviews.

During the enactment of *Hansel and Gretel*, Tasha focused on issues of food, both through restriction and in abundance. As the story unfolded, Tasha, as both Hansel and Gretel, was careful to save the slice of bread that her Stepmother gave them. She then left the breadcrumbs as the story suggests, only to find that the Bird had eaten them. Once the siblings find themselves truly lost in the woods, Tasha actually hid alongside the office refrigerator. Then they followed the Bird to the gingerbread house and once again she began to eat.

COMMENTARY 16

Tasha explored these conflicting issues regarding restriction and abundance because of her own inner struggle to achieve a balance. As narrator, the therapist had difficulty thinking of enough descriptive terms to keep up with Tasha's devouring of the gingerbread house. 'Story, then, is a form of drama that examines, among other things, the often paradoxical relationship between the narrator and the characters and events narrated' (Landy 1993, p.31). As narrator, the therapist must be aware of the significance of the events being narrated as they affect or are affected by the characters. The therapist was careful to use pauses, in case she would want to stop eating, but she didn't.

Narrator / Therapist: And Hansel and Gretel went over to the gingerbread house and they began to eat.

Hansel and Gretel / Tasha: [*She begins to eat.*]

Narrator: They ate gingerbread [*pause*] and ate candy ribbons and they ate candy canes and they ate M&Ms [*pause*] and they ate peanut brittle and they ate more gingerbread and they had more peanut brittle and they had more sugar cane.

Hansel / Gretel: [*Continues to eat without stopping.*]

Narrator: [*Pause*] And they had gumdrops, yellow and blue and green and orange and they ate and they ate [*pause*] and they ate that gingerbread house.

COMMENTARY 17

Once again Tasha ravished the candy house, bit by bit. The therapist noticed that as she ate her head was turned slightly away, as if she knew it was something that she shouldn't be doing, both literally and figuratively.

As soon as the protagonists entered into the Witch's house, they sat down and ate again! This time it was a lunch prepared by the Witch who was pretending to be a kind old lady. As the story unfolded, the Witch tried to fatten Hansel who was in the cage, just as Gretel ended up pushing the Witch into the oven.

COMMENTARY 18

The story of Hansel and Gretel is about dire need. There is not enough food for the children. This appeared to represent Tasha's own struggle with her restrictive diet and the serious, life-threatening implications should she falter. The Witch took full advantage of the children's voracious appetites with every intention of devouring them. Tasha must not succumb to this daily temptation. This is a further indication that the issue of fear of bodily harm or death is being explored, as when the Witch is planning to bake and eat Hansel. This is in addition to the issue of loss of control, which relates directly to Tasha's need to control her cravings.

As the next few sessions evolved, Tasha continued to express herself through the dramatherapy sessions. Tasha's ability to express herself had progressed as the dramatherapy sessions unfolded. She chose make-up each time and explored a few new stories. She appeared to be very relaxed during the next few sessions. As the gingerbread cookie, she called out 'Nanny, nanny, pooh, pooh' whenever anyone tried to catch and eat her. Then she would sing out, 'You can't catch me, I'm a little gingerbread.' She actually became the 'Wolf' (fox) just in time to gobble herself (gingerbread cookie) up.

COMMENTARY 19

During that particular session, she had high sugars and wasn't able to play outside with the other children. She had to stay in a little red wagon, only to watch. Yet through drama she could (pretend to) run like the gingerbread cookie while everyone wanted to devour her, only to devour herself by becoming the antagonist at the very end of the story. Up until now, she had only played the parts of the protagonists, but she couldn't resist the opportunity to eat a cookie, if only figuratively. Paradoxically, in doing so she destroyed herself.

Other children (Case 4) have also referred to the Fox in The Gingerbread Man *as a Wolf. The Wolf is an all-powerful and universal antagonist. The fox is not as familiar to classic literature. In addition, Tasha may be substituting the Wolf from* Little Red Riding Hood *for the fox, whom she had previously faced. It is significant that Tasha was able to avoid being the helpless cookie by instantaneously becoming the victorious Wolf/Fox. In doing so, she was able to address her oral fixation. It was during the eighth session that Tasha introduced a new character. It was the role of death.*

Session #8: Jack and the Beanstalk

During the eighth session, Tasha selected the story of *Jack and the Beanstalk*, and the character of Jack. Tasha looked through the drama bag and took out a wooden skeleton stick-puppet. She placed it on the desk where the therapist sat, and began a dialogue.

Therapist:	You want to play puppets?
Tasha:	Is this a wooden puppet?
Therapist:	He lost his head, though. [*Puppet's head had accidentally been broken off while in the bag.*]
Tasha:	Huh…he hasn't lost his head.
Therapist:	[*Laughs*] Yes, he did. It's in the bag, somewhere.
Tasha:	Hmmm.
Therapist:	He lost his head.
Tasha:	I know where his head is.
Therapist:	Where?
Tasha:	[*Points to the protruding stick where the head used to be.*] Right here.

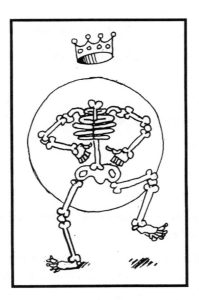

Figure 4.5 You could hear the rattling bones of the madly dancing Skeleton (illustration by Laurence Muleh 2001)

Therapist:	Oh, I see. I see what you mean.
Tasha:	Ahh. [*Pulls puppet's string to make his arms and legs dance.*] Ya, ya, ya. Here are his hands. Right here. He's a skeleton.
Therapist:	He's a skeleton, isn't he?
Skeleton/Tasha:	Hi! I am a skeleton. Oh, look at that…a tape recorder. Is it on?
Therapist:	It is on.
Skeleton:	Oooh, look at this tape recorder. Ain't it so nice?
Therapist:	Why thank you, Skeleton. I'm glad you like the tape recorder.
Skeleton:	I didn't come from this world. I don't know what's in this.
Therapist:	I don't know. I think you lost your head.
Skeleton:	I did not. I'm a skeleton.
Therapist:	Ooh, well if you're a skeleton, where's the person?
Skeleton:	He died a long time ago.
Therapist:	He did?
Skeleton:	And that's why I'm in his bones.
Therapist:	Well, it's a pleasure to meet you.
Skeleton:	I'm not leavin' yet.
Therapist:	Well it's a pleasure to have you here. Are you going to do the story with us today?
Skeleton:	No.
Therapist:	Oh.
Skeleton:	I just came to visit.
Therapist:	Would you like to watch the story, and you could be an audience?
Skeleton:	Yeah, hold on. [*Makes skeleton's arms and legs move.*] Hold on here, I have to go back to the grave.
Therapist:	Oohh, well come back and see us again.
Skeleton:	I'm coming back.

Therapist:	Are you a nice skeleton or a scary skeleton?
Skeleton:	I'm a scary skeleton.
Therapist:	Ahh. [*The skeleton attacks.*]
Skeleton:	I am going to bite you.
Therapist:	What?
Skeleton:	I am going to bite you.
Therapist:	Don't you dare. I'll call Tasha. Ahh. [*The skeleton pretends to bite the therapist.*] Help!
Skeleton:	Hold on. I'll be back, I said. [*Pause*] Hello.
Therapist:	Which skeleton are you?
Skeleton:	The nice mean nice.
Therapist:	Which one?
Skeleton:	The nice skeleton.
Therapist:	Well, you won't believe it but there was a mean skeleton here that tried to scare me. In fact, he did. Now he's gone.
Skeleton:	Hold on, hold on. [*Pause*] Hello. [*Attacks*]
Therapist:	Ahhhh! [*Being attacked by the 'mean' skeleton.*]
Skeleton:	I am the mean one. Ah, yah, ah, yah, yah.
Therapist:	Go away.
Skeleton:	OK. That's it. Let's do your movie. OK. I'm going to leave.
Therapist:	Good grief.
Tasha:	That was called the scary story. You gotta write that one down.

COMMENTARY 20

Tasha's introduction of the skeleton proved to be a turning point in the dramatherapy sessions. During this, the eighth session, for the first time she took on a role other than the protagonists from every previous session. This was the beginning of a new pattern and a new exploration for Tasha. The invocation of the role of death is clearly significant to Tasha's everyday life. According to Landy:

> *The therapeutic actor, like the theatrical actor, is given permission to move in and out of two contiguous realities: that of the imagination, the source of unconscious imagery, and that of the everyday, the domain of grounded daily existence. (Landy 1993, p.46)*

Tasha's exploration of death through this unconscious imagery represents an unmet need for expression of this issue as it relates to her daily existence. In Landy's taxonomy of roles (1993), the role type of death is examined. The quality of the role of death is described as 'one of the earliest roles personified in ancient dramatic rituals. As a type, death is threatening and terrifying, the incarnation of non-being' (Landy 1993, p.240).

In terms of physical qualities, the role of death, as is symbolized by the skeleton, is ugly and ageless. The skeleton indicates the result of poor and declining health. Tasha's portrayal of death is deceitful, alienating, and aggressive. By invoking such a scary and terrifying role, Tasha is able to begin to face her fears. Impending death is a reality that chronically ill children face every day. By creating an alternative or sub-role, that of the 'nice' skeleton, Tasha was able to quickly distance herself from the dark side. However, the 'nice' skeleton actually became the 'mean' skeleton's attempt to deceive.

Because death is so threatening, Tasha chose to portray death through a puppet rather than with her preferred use of make-up. This is because the puppet is safer and a more distanced choice for Tasha. The style of the role of death is presentational, as is further defined in Landy's taxonomy of roles. The wooden skeleton stick-puppet had movable arms and legs that were manipulated by a string. This gave the illusion of rattling bones. Tasha's role of death was therefore explored in a presentational manner, through this stylized skeleton.

The therapist suggested integrating this role into the fairy tale itself, but she was not yet ready to do so. At this point the role of death is not within a story but exists outside the story. This distances the role's essence. This is necessary for Tasha in initially creating such a life-threatening role. Tasha's anger was expressed again through the skeleton's attempt to bite and devour. Yet, this time it was directed at the therapist who was not in a role, other than that of therapist. Her anger may have been in part because she hadn't been seen in two weeks because of her partial hospital program schedule variation. The role of death appeared to relate to her life-threatening illness. The skeleton's angry biting related to her own anger and frustration in dietary restrictions, with the overwhelming consequences should she not abide.

According to Chetwynd (1982, p.114), a madly dancing skeleton is a 'macabre figure of death…though the figures are often fascinating to children.' Like the skeleton, the staff social worker describes Tasha as being 'very brittle' and 'shaky.' But, in addition to the brittle and shaky skeleton's representation of death lies the duality of good versus evil. Tasha has differentiated one good skeleton from one mean skeleton, although a single puppet represents both. Young children with a chronic illness such as diabetes 'often attribute the illness or the pain associated with their treatment to punishment for being bad' (O'Dougherty and Brown 1990, p.337). Tasha may have been projecting that 'bad' self into the role of the bad skeleton.

After the skeleton had left, Tasha and the therapist proceeded to prepare to act out the selected story for that session, *Jack and the Beanstalk*. But after just a few minutes of planning, the skeleton returned:

Tasha:	Here we are…
Skeleton / Tasha:	[*Deepens her voice*] Hey, how ya' doing? Huh? How ya' doing? How ya' doin'?
Therapist:	Uh, how are ya doing?
Skeleton:	Remember me? The mean one?
Therapist:	Oh, no! We're planning to do make-up.
Skeleton:	I love make-up. That's why I came here, to eat the make-up.
Therapist:	Oohh.
Skeleton:	Can you put some on me? Would you? Could you? Please, I'll be nice.
Therapist:	Well, we were going to put make-up on Tasha.
Skeleton:	Who's that?
Therapist:	She's my friend, right here.
Skeleton:	I don't see her?
Therapist:	Is that because you don't have any eyes?
Skeleton:	I do have eyes. And that's why I'm going to bite you.
Therapist:	Aahhh…no…Ow! [*Skeleton attacks.*]

Skeleton:	Bye-bye.
Therapist:	Bye.

COMMENTARY 21

The skeleton returns because of the power and significance of the role of death. The function of death is '...to claim the lives of mortals' (Landy 1993, p.240). This role can be scary for a 7-year-old girl, as can the reality that her chronic illness could result in her own death. This time he wanted to eat the make-up. He promised to be nice if he could wear the make-up. This reiterates the premise that 'if I'm good, I should be given privileges, not punishments.' Tasha's invoking of the good and bad skeleton also suggested an attempt to explore the counterparts of a single role. She was actually splitting the role of death into its opposites in an effort to seek balance.

During this session, Tasha continued to be more interactive than before. She appeared to be more expressive and motivated. She referred to her favorite part of Jack and the Beanstalk as 'when he fell off the tree.' This translated to when the Giant plunged off the beanstalk and died. Once again she was exploring the issue of death. Death is a significant issue in fairy tales, however, and is often self-chosen (Heuscher 1974). An example is the Gingerbread Man who runs from antagonist to antagonist, while narrowly escaping death each time. Then he ends up on the Fox's nose, only to be gobbled. This is considered a self-inflicted death for the cookie. Tasha had not only chosen to dramatize death-related scenes, but moreover added the skeleton, or death character, to the sessions. Just as death in fairy tales is usually chosen, Tasha chose to explore death through the dramatizations. Faced with a life-threatening illness, Tasha chose to explore death through her role-playing. The issue of fear of bodily harm or death became Tasha's focus for the remainder of her dramatherapy sessions.

Session #9: Little Red Riding Hood

During the ninth session Tasha returned to her favorite story, *Little Red Riding Hood.* This time, however, she was prepared to be the antagonist; in this case, the Wolf. She selected the black, furry mask to wear and requested to act out the whole story. 'I'm mean this time,' she said. Then she added, 'I'm dressed in black already.' This referred to her own outfit, which happened to be all black that day.

As the story unfolded, the Wolf (Tasha) was able to discover from Little Red Riding Hood (therapist) where the Grandmother lived. From there the Wolf proceeded to devour first the Grandmother, and as the story goes, then Little Red Riding Hood. For the first time Tasha was able not only to take on the role of the antagonist, but also to take on a role with an all-consuming and insatiable appetite.

COMMENTARY 22

According to Thomas (1989): 'The Wolf embodies the threat of all asocial, barbaric, unconscious, devouring powers... his appetite is bestial.' As the Wolf, Tasha can devour entire human beings. She is finally able to take on the role that actually personifies bodily harm and death. She is no longer seeking the comfort of the role of the protagonist, but has become the very essence of this oral creature symbolic of the untamed.

Once the Huntsman chopped the Wolf, saving Little Red Riding Hood and Grandmother, the story ended, yet only temporarily.

Therapist:	[*After the initial dramatization.*] Now then, what was your favorite part of the story?
Tasha:	Ummm...the end.
Therapist:	And what do you like best about the end of the story?
Tasha:	I don't know.
Therapist:	But you liked the end best? [*Pause, she nods.*] Well, in the end the Wolf ate Little Red, the Wolf ate Grandmother and then the Hunter...the Hunter came in and chopped the Wolf. And then what happened to the Wolf then?
Tasha:	The Wolf? The Wolf came back to life. He was an Angel then.
Therapist:	An Angel then?
Tasha:	But nobody can see him.
Therapist:	Ohh, I see.

The story in Tasha's mind didn't end with herself as the Wolf dying, as in the original fairy tale. Nor was the story to end, as in earlier sessions, with the therapist as the Wolf dying. So, with a few moments remaining the therapist asked her:

Therapist:	Do you want to do the story of the Angel Wolf?
Tasha:	Yeah.
Therapist:	Let's do the Angel Wolf.
Tasha:	Do you know how to do it?
Therapist:	Uh huh.
Tasha:	Huh?
Therapist:	Yes, do you?
Tasha:	No.
Therapist:	All right, we're going to do the end. Who do you want to be?
Tasha:	The Wolf.
Therapist:	OK. And the Wolf becomes the Angel Wolf.
Tasha:	Yes. Here's the Angel. Hmmm, what should I...like that [*She sets up with the black, furry mask and king's crown, then makes sure that the tape recorder is working.*]
Narrator/Therapist:	This is the story of what happens in *Little Red Riding Hood* with a new ending; it's called 'The Angel Wolf.' As our story continues, the Wolf had just gobbled up Grandmother and Little Red Riding Hood. And just then the Huntsman appeared.
Tasha:	OK [*into the microphone of the tape recorder*]. This was on channel 39, which is the kids' channel. Bye. Change back to channel 39 in one minute.
Little Red/Therapist:	Help, help.
Huntsman/Therapist:	Who is it that needs help? Where's Grandmother?
Tasha:	I'm not...you can't see me.
Narrator/Therapist:	OK. So the Wolf got chopped up [*chop, chop*] and the Wolf was gone. So the Huntsman said to the Mother...
Huntsman/Therapist:	Oh, don't worry, Little Red is fine, and don't you worry, Grandmother is fine now. Don't worry, Mother.

Narrator / Therapist: So, Mother and the Huntsman and Little Red and Grandmother lived very happily ever after. But, Mother said...

Mother / Therapist: What became of the Wolf?

Huntsman / Therapist: Well, I'm sorry to tell you this but the Wolf was so mean, and after the Wolf gobbled up Little Red and after the Wolf ate Grandmother, we had to chop up the Wolf, and now the little Wolf is gone from earth and has become an Angel Wolf.

Tasha: Well, I'm not really an Angel right now. Yeah, I'm a Wolf now and I feel like gobbling you up.

Therapist: Aaahhh! [*Is attacked by Wolf.*] No. Don't do it! How did the Wolf come back? We thought you were dead.

Wolf / Tasha: [*Puts hat on.*] You can't see me with this hat on.

Therapist: Hey, where did she go? The Wolf is gone. Don't worry, you're just seeing things. The Wolf is gone. The Wolf is dead.

Wolf / Tasha: I'm right here.

Therapist: Oohh, where did that Wolf go? I can't believe my eyes. The Wolf's there and then the Wolf's gone.

Wolf / Tasha: I'm right here.

Therapist: Please, Mr Wolf, why did you gobble us up?

Wolf / Tasha: Uhh. It's just a kid's cartoon.

Therapist: Ooh, it's just a cartoon for kids.

COMMENTARY 23

When Tasha, as the Wolf, wore the hat (king's crown), no one could see her. When the crown was removed, she could be seen. A game of 'now-you-see-me, now-you-don't,' or peek-a-boo, ensued. This playful interaction is normally explored during the early developmental stages with one's mother. It is considered a way in which a healthy child makes sure that mother is still going to be there during the individuation process: '[it is] at the critical stage of the separation of not-me from the me, when the establishment of an autonomous self is at the initial stage' (Winnicott 1971, p.110).

The session continues:

Wolf/Tasha:	Do you see me?
Therapist:	I hear you but I don't see you.
Wolf/Tasha:	I'm invisible.
Therapist:	How is it possible, that you're invisible?
Tasha:	Do you see this king's hat?
Therapist:	I don't see anything.
Tasha:	You can see it but you can't see me.
Therapist:	I see the king's crown, but I don't see you. What does that mean?
Tasha:	Do you see this little box? [*Holds a miniature tape box.*]
Therapist:	Yes, it's floating in air. I don't see anyone holding it.
Wolf/Tasha:	Do you see it…the paper out?
Therapist:	Yeah, I do.
Wolf/Tasha:	Hold on. Do you see that?
Therapist:	Yes, I do [*pause*]. But, tell me, can you hear me?
Wolf/Tasha:	I can hear everything that you say.
Therapist:	Are you really dead?
Wolf/Tasha:	Probably, I can come back if you want me to.
Therapist:	Well, will you gobble us up again?
Wolf/Tasha:	Only if you don't fix a cake for pretend.
Therapist:	A cake?
Wolf/Tasha:	If you fix a cake then I won't gobble you up.
Therapist:	Oh, we'll fix you a cake.
Wolf/Tasha:	Well, you better have it ready and I'll set my clock and it's on one minute and it better be done in one minute.
Therapist:	OK.
Wolf:	Time is running up.
Therapist:	[*Prepares a cake.*]
Wolf:	Your time is running out.

Therapist:	[*Hums while baking.*]
Wolf:	And it better have chocolate on it, too!
Therapist:	[*Continues to hum while baking.*]
Wolf:	Time out.
Therapist:	Where's the Wolf?
Wolf:	I'm not back yet.
Therapist:	Would you, could you? Would you like some chocolate cake, our friend the Wolf?
Wolf:	I'm eating your hand right now.
Therapist:	I made you the chocolate cake like you asked. You promised that you wouldn't gobble us up if we made you cake. Maybe you'll be our friend.
Wolf:	Never listen to wolves. Never. [*The Wolf proceeds to gobble up the Huntsman and Little Red.*]

COMMENTARY 24

The only way the Wolf will come back from the dead and be good (i.e., not gobble people) was with the promise of a chocolate cake. Ironically, a chocolate cake would be life threatening for Tasha. Yet, if she could have this temptation she wouldn't feel the urge to devour entire human beings. When the therapist (as the collective protagonists) does as she (the Wolf) wishes, they are punished by death for submitting. For Tasha, who is insulin dependent, she must never listen to the wolves of temptation. Never, because as her story ended, so did the lives of the 'good guys.' Tasha knew the consequences if she were to give in to them. She proceeded to title the story as if it were a television show, called 'Are You Afraid of the Dark?'

Session #10: The Three Little Pigs

Tasha was hiding under the desk in the therapy room during the beginning of the tenth and last session.

Therapist:	Oh, I don't know where she is? Well, I'll tell you what I'll do. I'll go outside the door, count to five and come back in, and maybe she'll be here. [*Therapist leaves momentarily, yet with the door ajar, and begins to count...*] One...two...three...four...five. [*Enters the room. Tasha*

remains hidden.] OK, I'm going to close my eyes and count to ten and when I open them Tasha will be here so we can do our story, especially since today is our last day. One...[*counts loudly*] ...two...three...four...five [*counts in rapid succession*] six, seven, eight, nine, ten. Where on earth? Come out, come out, wherever you are...apples, peaches, pumpkin pie, come out, come out, wherever you are. Uh, oh, the chair is moving and there's nobody in it. How are you going to explain that one [*Tasha continues to move the chair, while remaining hidden under the desk.*] Tasha, come out. Are you in here?

Tasha:	[*Mumbles faintly from under the desk.*]
Therapist:	What?
Tasha:	[*Mumbles inaudibly.*]
Therapist:	Where?
Tasha:	I am the bear. [*Holds out a stuffed bear.*]
Therapist:	Oh, Tasha, is this you?
Tasha:	Yeah.
Therapist:	All right, I'll put you right here in the chair. [*Places bear in chair.*] Are you ready for drama?

During the next few minutes, all of the therapist's comments are directed to the stuffed bear in the chair. Tasha provides the voice in selecting the story of *The Three Little Pigs* and the role of the 'Brick Pig.' While remaining hidden, she selects a mask for the teddy bear to wear. Then she finally emerges.

COMMENTARY 25

The therapist allows Tasha to remain hidden and plays along with the patient's temporary need to take control through avoidance. Although the therapist wanted to start the session, it was important to be aware of the patient's needs. This interaction is a further extension of her previous hide-and-seek behavior. The fact that it has manifested itself during the last few sessions and has increased in longevity is significant. This enactment is also emerging as a pattern within the dramatizations themselves. This suggests the child's continued exploration of individuation, as well as the issue of separation anxiety.

Tasha selects the masks and props for the story.

Tasha:	I have an ending for this one too. It's going to be like the Angel one.
Therapist:	Oh, yes, the Angel story.
Tasha:	I need the king's hat. I need the king's hat. You're going to be pink [*referring to a pink pig mask*]. OK? I'm the king and you got to get your mask on. Hold on. I like the Wolf.

Tasha proceeded to set up for the story. Tasha was to be a king and a wolf. The therapist was to be a pig. She had become very verbal over the last few sessions. She was able to complete entire sentences. Tasha appeared to be motivated and knew exactly how the story was to unfold. She was singing as she set up.

Narrator/Tasha:	This is the story of…what [*to herself*] …*The Three Little Pigs*. And this is the channel 12 news and I am a Wolf.
Therapist:	Are you ready?
Tasha:	[*Sings*] So, you see my nose, you see my eyes. You know that flies…bye.
Therapist:	Ready?
Tasha:	Hold on, hold on, do do do do do da do [*sings*]. Action, camera, lights…
Narrator/Therapist:	[*As the story unfolded, Tasha took on the role of the Brick Pig as she had originally selected.*] But the smartest of all pigs worked very, very hard to make the strongest house. And it took days and nights and nights and days and finally… [*as therapist*] who should be the Wolf?
Tasha:	I will.
Therapist:	So, one day the Wolf came along and saw a little house of straw.
Wolf/Tasha:	Knock! Knock!
Pig/Therapist:	Who is it?
Wolf:	Knock, knock. Let me in, let me in.

Pig:	Not by the hair of my chinny chin chin.
Wolf:	Then I'll blow your house down.
Pig:	Ah, no.
Wolf:	[*She huffs and puffs and blows down the house.*]

COMMENTARY 26

The story repeats according to the original tale. Tasha has taken on the roles of both the Wolf and the Brick Pig. She is now portraying both the antagonist and the protagonist. This is, for Tasha, one way to maintain control. Identifying with the hero-protagonist suggests that each of us is our own life's hero (Thomas 1989). Tasha plays the role of the smarter and older Pig, which according to the original tale is the hero:

> *The protagonist / hero is both the force which generates all other characters and actions, an axial being around whom they revolve – the squarely central point around which the tale's perfect circle spins. This constitutes the narrative's locus and focus, the protagonist possesses a power which speaks to one's intellect, emotions and imagination. (Thomas 1989, p.62)*

The hero represents the child's own plight. Yet, Tasha also plays the role of the antagonist, which she wasn't wanting to or able to portray in any of the earliest sessions. The Wolf is excessively greedy and lives on its prey. There is never any sympathy for the Wolf, who is found to be deserving of whatever punishment he receives. Tasha's need to explore both opposing forces at once allows her to examine her own contradicting turmoil, while maintaining some sense of security. By exploring the roles of both the Wolf and Little Red simultaneously, Tasha was working towards a balance by invoking counter-roles. The role of the Wolf and the role of Little Red are opposites. The Wolf represents all that is dark and evil, whereas Little Red is all that is pure and pristine. The role of Little Red represents hope, which counters the Wolf's impending doom.

As the protagonist, she is able to preserve the rationale and safety of good sense, while at the same time becoming a murderous beast of prey (Rowland 1973). She is finally able to become, and therefore confronts, her own unconscious and terrifying fears. By exploring the roles of both protagonist and antagonist in the same story, Tasha can delve into her own conflicting battle of opposing forces that she faces on a daily basis.

Wolf/ Tasha:	Knock, knock.
Pig/ Therapist:	Who is it?
Wolf:	It's the Wolf.
Pig:	Go away.
Wolf:	Why?
Pig:	You cannot come in and gobble us up.
Wolf:	Hold on, I'm not the Wolf.
Pig:	Oh, who is it?
Wolf:	I'm your friend.
Pig:	Oh.
Wolf:	And I am the Wolf.
Pig:	You cannot come in.
Wolf:	All right.
Pig:	The Wolf's at the door. The Wolf's at the door.
Wolf:	Yes, the Wolf is here.

The therapist best serves the needs of the patients by going along with their story line. Even though the therapist in-role knows it was the Wolf, she must follow the patient's logic and suspend her disbelief. As Tasha explored this situation, she created several different ways in which the Wolf could achieve access into the Pig's house. She said, 'I'm not the Wolf, I'm your friend.' So the therapist (Pig) talked to the oldest and smartest Pig (also played by Tasha) and got her approval to let the 'friend' in. The Wolf, who was disguised as a bear, got in and requested scrambled eggs and pig's feet for dinner. This suggested to the Pigs that he might in fact be the Wolf after all. Then Tasha knocked on the door again, this time stating, 'I'm a friendly Wolf.' So, once again the Wolf was allowed in, with the approval of the oldest Pig (Tasha). This time the Wolf requested 'pig soup.' The third time, the Wolf got access into the house by requesting a visit with his sister and brother. Once she gained entrance, she revealed that she was not a Pig, but the Wolf, and proceeded to eat everyone. She revealed her true identity. Then she knocked on the door again, this time entering and asking to be shot.

Wolf:	Could you shoot me?
Pig:	Are you the big bad Wolf?
Wolf:	Yeah.
Pig:	[*Shoots.*]
Wolf:	I'm not dead.
Pig:	[*Shoots again.*]
Wolf:	I'm not dead.
Pig:	[*Shoots again.*]
Wolf:	Shoot my ears or my eyes. I'm not dead [*pause*] I'm in heaven, so you can't see me.
Pig:	Oh, what is going on here?
Wolf:	You cannot see anything.
Pig:	Where did you go?
Wolf:	I'm up in heaven.
Pig:	I can't see you.
Wolf:	I'm way up. I'm up, too, so you can't see me. [*As time ran out in the session she explained that everybody died as the story ended.*] Well, we got to finish you up. Where did the spoon go? OK, come here [*to pig*]. I'm going to eat you. [*Eats pig.*] Here, have some food.
Tasha:	[*Referring to Wolf*] This thing could eat anything, and now it's trying to eat you.

COMMENTARY 27

The therapist must accept the patient's rendition of the story, because the ability to create improvisationally is one way that the unconscious is able to express unresolved conflicts. During this exploration, Tasha repeatedly reenacts the scene where the Wolf tries to enter the Pig's house. Each time she finds a way to get into the house, it is herself as the oldest and smartest Pig that accepts and approves of her own entrance as the Wolf. The Wolf has one motivation and one goal, that is to eat the forbidden Pigs. She, in a sense, is giving herself permission to do the 'bad' thing. As the Wolf, she hints of her true motivation by requesting 'pig soup' and 'pig's feet' for dinner. As the story line climaxes, she eats all of the Pigs and in the next moment asks to be shot. She then, after minimal resistance, dies and goes to heaven, where she still devours Pigs. Because the Wolf succumbs to his temptation and untamed appetite, he consequently dies. Unlike the original fairy tale, whereas the Pigs outsmart the Wolf, this Wolf gets his wish but dies because of it. If Tasha were to give in to her untamed appetite, it would be life threatening. If she were to give herself the approval (like the oldest and smartest Pig) to devour all that she wanted (like the Wolf) the consequences would be dire. Tasha was able to explore this inner turmoil through her dramatization of this fairy tale.

Discussion

During the initial dramatherapy sessions, Tasha presented herself as withdrawn, shy, and minimally verbal. Her medical chart described her as depressed, anxious, and inattentive. The medical records also indicated that Tasha was below average to borderline in her cognitive, academic and memory skills. Although Tasha was, at first, somewhat limited in her ability to express herself, she progressed greatly over the ten sessions. As the case study indicates, Tasha was initially withdrawn, yet she was empowered by her involvement in the dramatizations.

A once withdrawn and seemingly depressed child became motivated, animated, and highly interactive. The quality of the role-playing evolved as is indicated by both the developments of the plots and dialogues, as well as her willingness to communicate. At first her dialogues contained simply a word or two, then her conversation began to flow. An ease came over Tasha as the dramatherapy sessions unfolded, which was combined with an earnest excitability. A personal transformation had evolved.

The stress measure (Antoni 1993) which was used in all cases as an observational tool, indicates an improvement in Tasha's stress level. Tasha's results indicate that almost all stress-related symptoms showed a marked reduction. This scale suggests that Tasha's stress was significantly reduced (see Appendix A). The three major sources of stress in chronically ill children, which have been cited as separation anxiety, loss of control, and fear of bodily harm or death, were pertinent issues in Tasha's dramatizations. All three stress-related issues were explored through the dramatherapy. As is indicated in the case study, the issue of separation anxiety was present in the earlier sessions, particularly within

Little Red Riding Hood going off into the woods and Hansel and Gretel being left in the woods. There is a great anxiety for Hansel and Gretel in facing sheer abandonment from their Stepmother and Father, as they're left alone in the woods to fend for themselves. Tasha explored both of these stories twice during the earlier sessions, and then focused on the issue of fear of loss of control, as it related to her restricted appetite.

As Tasha vicariously devoured the gingerbread house in the roles of Hansel and Gretel, and then proceeded to devour herself as the gingerbread cookie, she was acting out the issue of fear of loss of control. Tasha must control her appetite daily because of her juvenile diabetes. As she explored this issue, the third and most significant stress-related factor began to emerge. Fear of bodily harm and more specifically, the issue of death, became a prominent issue and overall theme of Tasha's dramatizations. The issue first presented itself as a fear of harm during the earlier sessions, when the Wolf was a threat. By the eighth session, it was the role of death that Tasha portrayed in the form of a skeleton. Then death was further examined as Tasha took on the role of the Wolf who proceeds to die and go to heaven. She actually explored her own mortality. The roles were both existent and non-existent. One minute the character was there and the next minute it was not. This pattern was repeated. Tasha's progressive enactment of all three stress-related issues indicates an expression of stressors within the dramatizations, therefore a reduction in stress due to this release.

Parent and staff interviews confirm the severity of Tasha's illness. According to the staff social worker: 'She's very brittle. Her sugar has broken down a lot, even if she doesn't eat' (JM, personal communication, September 16 1997). Both the hospital staff and her mother stated that stress does play a part in Tasha's chronic illness. According to Tasha's primary nurse, stress increases Tasha's blood sugar. Therefore, a reduction in stress could benefit Tasha's medical condition.

When asked whether stress influenced her child's condition, Tasha's mother answered, 'I don't know. I know it does for me, so it must be for her. Kids don't really tell you. I'll ask, but she doesn't really speak.' This is another indication that Tasha is relatively non-verbal regarding her feelings towards her chronic illness. Her mother proceeded to state that Tasha's 'coping was better' since the dramatherapy sessions (Mrs S, personal communication, September 22 1997). The staff nurse concluded that Tasha really seemed to enjoy drama. She considered Tasha to be 'mild mannered, quiet and happy...not angry' (ML, personal communication, October 4 1997). This does indicate a change from the initial medical notes that described her as being depressed and impulsive. Overall, the interviews confirmed that Tasha's illness was exacerbated by stress, and that she liked the drama sessions. Her coping skills appeared to have improved, which may indicate a reduction in stress.

The Children's Manifest Anxiety Scale – Revised (CMAS-R) was administered as both a pre- and post-test. Tasha's pre-test score was 17, which is above the average score of 13.84. Tasha's post-test score was 14, which is very near the average, and indicates a reduction in anxiety. According to the CMAS-R, Tasha's stress and anxiety level were reduced from an above-average level to an average level (see Appendix A).

Based on clinical observation, stress measures and assessments, as well as the documented case study, it appears as though Tasha's stress level was reduced. There didn't appear to be an observable change in her medical condition, based on the data as presented. However, it appears that Tasha's stress level was reduced, particularly through the self-expression and the communication of significant issues. Such a minimally verbal and supposedly low functioning child may not otherwise have been able to explore such issues.

Six-Month Follow-Up

According to Tasha's primary nurse, her medical condition has improved over the past six months since the dramatherapy treatment (ML, personal communication, March 23 1998). Tasha is being considered for discharge from the hospital program by the next school year. Because her sugar levels are not completely under control, Tasha may have future medical problems resulting from her juvenile diabetes. However, not only has her medical condition improved, but behaviorally Tasha, who was always considered to be very shy, is now more outgoing with classmates (DS, personal communication, March 23 1998).

Transcript of selected session

Tasha: Selected Session #9 (9/9/97)

Therapist:	Today we are here with Tasha and Miss Carol.
Tasha:	I want to play something different.
Therapist:	Of course, oh you know what – before we go we have to do our questionnaire.
Tasha:	What's that?
Therapist:	Remember, it is the question and answer part? Do you want to do it first or before you leave?
Tasha:	Before we leave.
Therapist:	OK, don't let me forget. What story would you like to pick?
Tasha:	Ummm.
Therapist:	Ummm. *Hansel and Gretel?*
Tasha:	No.
Therapist:	*Jack and the Beanstalk?*
Tasha:	No.
Therapist:	*Little Red Riding Hood?*
Tasha:	Yes.
Therapist:	*Gingerbread Man, Three Little Pigs?*
Tasha:	*Red Riding Hood.*
Therapist:	Little Red? Now would you like me to tell you the story or do you already know it?
Tasha:	We already know it.
Therapist:	All right. Now for today if you could be anyone in *Little Red Riding Hood* who would you be?
Tasha:	Red Riding Hood.
Therapist:	And would you like to use anything in the bag?
Tasha:	What's *Little Red Riding Hood?* I forgot that.

Therapist:	It's the one where Little Red Riding Hood goes to visit Grandmother who's sick, and she goes along the path and the Wolf jumps out and says, 'Where are you going?'
Tasha:	I want to be the Wolf this time.
Therapist:	And the Wolf says — remember the Wolf says, 'Grandmother, what big ears you have.'
Tasha:	You've gotta say that.
Therapist:	OK, you be the Wolf and I'll be Little Red. Oh, my goodness, don't tell me. Now, do you remember this story? Yeah, I know you're trying to scare me with that mask and it worked. It's very scary.
Tasha:	Very scary.
Therapist:	All right. Let's begin.
Tasha:	Look at the bear — look!
Therapist:	Yes, are you ready for the story? Are you going to be the Wolf?
Tasha:	Yeah. But you're not telling it yet.
Therapist:	We'll do it together.
Tasha:	Oooh! Somebody broke it.
Therapist:	Ahhh, well we'll have to sew and cut it.
Tasha:	Cut it. Where's the scissors?
Therapist:	That I don't know. We'll fix it.
Tasha:	Have you been in here a long time?
Therapist:	Oh, here's scissors.
Tasha:	I've been here a lot of times.
Therapist:	Oh yes, you're doing very good!
Tasha:	Do you play on that computer?
Therapist:	No.
Tasha:	'Cause you don't know whose it is?
Therapist:	Right.
Tasha:	You're allowed to play on it, I bet.

Therapist:	Probably. Now you want me to help you get that on?
Tasha:	Probably.
Therapist:	Can you get it?
Tasha:	Nope.
Therapist:	It's velcro. Does it stick?
Tasha:	Yeah.
Therapist:	OK – here we go.
Tasha:	Hold on, hold on – I'm not ready yet. I'm mean this time, I'm going to be real mean.
Therapist:	I bet.
Tasha:	Hold on.
Therapist:	Because that Wolf is a mean Wolf.
Tasha:	Hold on.
Therapist:	OK, take your time. What part of the story did you want to do? The whole story or the part with the Wolf?
Tasha:	The whole story. Hold on – hold on, let's make the forest look real mean.
Therapist:	Yeah, I'll say.
Mother / Therapist:	Little Red! Little Red! Listen to me, dear. Your Grandmother is sick. No, no – it's just a cold really but I want you to take this basket of goodies to her and that'll make her feel much, much better. But don't talk to strangers and stay on the path please.
Little Red / Therapist:	Yes, Mother, I'll take the goodies to Grandmother. I'll do just as you say. Goodbye, Mama.
	And Little Red went through the woods, 'Tra la la la, tra la la, I'm off to Grandmother's house. Tra la la la, tra la la, I'm off to Grandmother's house. Tra la la la la la, nobody will bother me.'
	So Little Red was going through the woods and all of a sudden, 'Whhhhh! What do you want?'
Wolf / Tasha:	Where are you going?
Little Red:	Why, I'm going to my Grandmother's house.

Wolf:	Where does she live?
Little Red:	Well, she lives right down the path past the third tree toward the very end in the little stone house.
Wolf:	Ohhh.
Little Red:	I'm bringing her these goodies.
Wolf:	What kind of goodies?
Little Red:	Well, there's some cookies and some pie.
Narrator / Therapist:	So Little Red went through the woods, not realizing she had just told the Wolf what she had.
Little Red:	Through the woods, 'Tra la la, tra la la, it's off to Grandmother's house I go. Tra la la, tra la la, it's off to Grandmother's house.'
Narrator / Therapist:	Well, before Little Red got there the Wolf came in and got rid of Grandmother, jumped into bed, pulled up the covers and waited for Little Red.
Tasha:	[*Laughing*]
Little Red:	And Little Red knocked on the door, 'Grandmother, are you here?'
Wolf:	Yes.
Little Red:	Where are you?
Wolf:	In the bed.
Little Red:	Oh, Grandmother. Grandmother! What big ears you have.
Wolf:	So I can hear.
Little Red:	Grandmother! What big eyes you have.
Wolf:	So I can see.
Little Red:	Grandmother! What big teeth you have.
Wolf:	To gobble you up.
Little Red:	Ehhhhhh!
Narrator / Therapist:	And the Wolf gobbled up Little Red and had already gobbled up Grandmother. But just then from out of the woods came a Huntsman who heard Little Red's cries.

Little Red:	Help! Help!
Huntsman:	'Oh, someone's in trouble, I'd better check.' So he went in the house. 'Ohhhhh! What did you do with Grandmother?'
Wolf:	I ate her up.
Huntsman:	Where's Little Red?
Wolf:	I ate her.
Huntsman:	Oh yeah! Watch this!

Narrator / Therapist: And he took the ax and was about to chop the Wolf. Chop – chop. And up pops Little Red and Grandmother.

Little Red and Grandmother: Oh thank you! Thank you! We're saved. The Wolf is gone. The Wolf is no more.

Therapist:	And that's the story of Little Red.
Tasha:	Yeah.
Therapist:	Did you like that story?
Tasha:	Yeah.
Therapist:	Did you like how it ended?
Tasha:	Em-hmmh.
Therapist:	So the Wolf got chopped up, I'm afraid.
Tasha:	Now we got three minutes.
Therapist:	We have more time now. That's a short story. Were you saying you would like the Wolf to come back at the end?
Tasha:	Um – probably.
Therapist:	So then what would happen?
Tasha:	The Wolf would come back.
Therapist:	Now what's your favorite part of the story?
Tasha:	The end.
Therapist:	And what do you like very best about the end of the story?
Tasha:	I don't know.

Therapist:	But you like the end best. In the end the Wolf ate Little Red. The Wolf ate Grandmother and then…
Tasha:	You forgot to draw the map. I know what we could play.
Therapist:	And then the Hunter came in and chopped up the Wolf and what happened to the Wolf then?
Tasha:	The Wolf came back alive. He was an Angel then.
Therapist:	He was an Angel then.
Tasha:	But nobody could see him.
Therapist:	Ohhhhh. I see. And Little Red and Grandmother and Mother and the Huntsman were very, very happy – and the Angel Wolf – lived very happily ever after. And that's the story.
Tasha:	Now you have to tell it on there. Not the whole story but the end of the story.
Therapist:	We changed the ending – didn't we?
Tasha:	I got something we could play since we got ooooh!
Therapist:	We still have a lot of time together but I want to ask you the questions. Remember we did this questionnaire once in the beginning of the summer.
Tasha:	OK, ask me now.
Therapist:	OK, here we go. Ready? Just yes or no answers. OK. [*Administers CMAS-R, The What I Think and Feel Test.*]
Tasha:	What's next?
Therapist:	Well – let me see. Well, we did our story.
Tasha:	We have to do another one.
Therapist:	I guess we have just enough time to clean up. Unless you want to do the end of the story. Do you want to do the story with the Angel Wolf?
Tasha:	Yeah.
Therapist:	Let's do the Angel Wolf.
Tasha:	Do you know how to do it?
Therapist:	Uh-huh.

Tasha:	Hah?
Therapist:	Yes, do you?
Tasha:	No.
Therapist:	All right. We're going to do the end.
Tasha:	We need a chair and we need an angel hat.
Therapist:	OK. Grab the angel hat from the bag. We've got just enough time to do the end of our story – the Angel Wolf.
Tasha:	OK.
Therapist:	Who are you going to be?
Tasha:	The Wolf.
Therapist:	OK and the Wolf becomes the Angel Wolf.
Tasha:	Yep and here's the angel. Who should this be – right there?
Therapist:	Let's flip it under here and see if it's…
Tasha:	It's like a tent though. Ooooh, we ain't getting record yet.
Therapist:	Oh it records either way. Don't worry.
Tasha:	Hold on. You got to tell the story about it.
Therapist:	This is the story of what happened to Little Red Riding Hood with a new ending. It's called the Angel Wolf. As our story continues, the Wolf had just gobbled up Grandmother and Little Red Riding Hood. And just then the Huntsman appeared.
Tasha:	This was on channel 39 which is 'Just for Kids' channel. Bye. Change back to channel 39 in one minute.
Little Red:	Help. Help.
Wolf:	Who is it that needs help?
Little Red:	Where's Grandmother?
Narrator/Therapist:	So the Wolf got chopped up. Chop-chop-chop. And the Wolf was gone.
Huntsman:	So the Huntsman said to Mother, 'Oh, don't worry – Little Red is fine and don't you worry. Grandmother's

fine now. Don't worry, Mother. And Mother and the
Huntsman and Little Red and Grandmother lived very
happily ever after.

Mother: But Mother said, 'What became of the Wolf?'
'We're sorry to tell you but the Wolf was so mean – well
after the Wolf gobbled up Little Red and after the Wolf
ate Grandmother we had to chop up the Wolf, and now
the little Wolf is gone from us and has become an Angel
Wolf.'

Tasha: Well I'm not really an Angel right now. Yeah I'm a Wolf
now and I feel like gobbling you up.

Mother: No, don't do it. How did the Wolf come back? I
thought you were dead.

Tasha: You can't see me with this hat on.

Mother: Don't worry, you were just seeing things. The Wolf is
gone. The Wolf is dead.

Tasha: I'm right here.

Mother: I can't believe my eyes, first the Wolf's dead, then the
Wolf's gone.

Tasha: I'm right here.

Mother: Please Mr Wolf, why did you...

Tasha: Emmm. It's just a kid's cartoon.

Mother: What?

Tasha: It's just a kid's cartoon.

Mother: Oh, is it the cartoon? For kids.

Tasha: Do you see me?

Therapist: Where did you go. I hear you but I don't see you.

Tasha: I'm invisible.

Therapist: How is that possible that you're invisible?

Tasha: Do you see this king's hat?
You can see it but you can't see me.

Therapist: I can see the king's crown but I don't see you.
What does that mean?

Tasha:	Can you see this little box?
Therapist:	Yes. It's floating in air. I don't see anyone holding it.
Tasha:	Do you see the paper out?
Therapist:	Yes, I do. [*Noise from microphone.*]
Tasha:	It's easy.
Therapist:	What does it mean?
Tasha:	You get walkie-talkies so they can hear you.
Therapist:	But tell me – can you hear me?
Tasha:	I can hear everything you say.
Therapist:	Are you really dead?
Tasha:	Probably. I could come back if you want me to.
Therapist:	Well, will you gobble those other people now?
Tasha:	Only if you don't fix a cake.
Therapist:	A cake.
Tasha:	If you fix a cake then I will not gobble you up.
Therapist:	Oh, we'll fix you a cake.
Tasha:	Well, you better have it ready, and I will set my clock and it's on one minute and it better be done in one minute.
Therapist:	OK. Bake the cake!
Tasha:	Time is running up.
Therapist:	[*Humming*]
Tasha:	Your time is running out. And it better have chocolate on it too!
Therapist:	[*Humming*]
Tasha:	Time's out. What do you want?
Therapist:	There's the Wolf.
Tasha:	I'm not back there.

Therapist:	Would you? Could you? Would you like some chocolate cake, my friend the Wolf?
Tasha:	Yeah. It's in your hand right now.
Therapist:	Here?
Tasha:	It's up there.
Therapist:	Where?
Tasha:	In the clouds.
Therapist:	Well, we made you the chocolate cake like you promised. You promised that you wouldn't gobble us up if we gave you cake. Maybe you'll be our friend?
Tasha:	Never listen to wolves. Never.
Therapist:	Uh-oh.
Tasha:	Ever.
Therapist:	What does that mean?
Tasha:	Who's that right there?
Therapist:	That's the Huntsman.
Tasha:	Tell him to come here or I'll get my walkie-talkie and he will come.
Therapist:	Oh, we just have one more minute.
Tasha:	OK.
Therapist:	Ahhh! No! Good story. Good story, Tasha. All right. We have just enough time. It's 1:30. All right. Let's put everything back in the bag. Tasha, that was a great twist on the story. That Wolf!!!
Tasha:	Oh, we didn't get under the house yet.
Therapist:	We can do that again Thursday. I have to get you back to your classroom.
Tasha:	Why we're leaving? Hold it. Hold it. That was the end of 39 and 'Are You Afraid of the Dark?' will be on when you get home. Have a lot of fun.

'Are You Afraid of the Dark?' And if it's not on, it will
be Nickelodeon. Channel Nickelodeon. Bye-bye.

Therapist: Bye-bye for now. Stay tuned for more of our story called
the Angel Wolf starring Tasha.

Our truest life is when we are in dreams awake.

Henry David Thoreau

Run, Run, as Fast as You Can't...

This case reflects how a child's emotional suffering and pain can easily
manifest itself by way of anger. Through Brandon's passion for acting,
he was able to work through some unresolved conflicts.

Background

Brandon is an 11-year-old boy with severe asthma. He was diagnosed at
age five. His asthma is triggered by colds, weather changes, pollen,
carpeting, and cigarette smoke (his father smokes). Because of severe
attacks that could not be controlled at home, Brandon was hospitalized
on five occasions, all in 1995 and 1996. His treatments include a
nebulizer breathing treatment that is administered three times a day,
blood tests, allergy shots, chest X-rays and up to seven different medications, including prednisone. The severity of Brandon's medical condition can lead to chest pain, headaches, stomach pain, and frequent
asthma attacks. Brandon has at least one asthma attack per week:

> Asthma, also described as reactive airway disease, is a common
> disorder whose basic symptoms are episodic attacks of chest tight-
> ness and wheezing. Physiologically, it is caused by dramatic, repeti-
> tive, intermittent inflammation and constriction of the airways.
> Asthma frequently begins in early childhood... (Mrazek 1993,
> p.194)

Severe asthma attacks, as in Brandon's case, can result in death.
Therefore, Brandon was admitted to this partial hospitalization

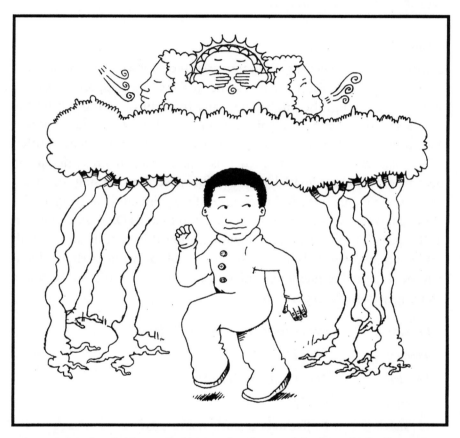

Figure 4.6 As the mischievous Cookie, Brandon discovered that he could finally run free (illustration by Laurence Muleh 2001)

program on January 1 1997 in order to monitor closely his chronic illness and to provide him with daily rigorous treatments. By attending school in this hospital program, Brandon was able to avoid a high absenteeism rate that had occurred during his attendance at his own school.

Description and Analysis

Session #1: Introduction

During our first meeting, Brandon presented himself as a somewhat defensive pre-adolescent with some reserve and apprehension. It appeared as though he might reject any thought of acting within the drama sessions. As the therapist explained to him what drama was, it was discovered that Brandon was the lead in his school play, entitled *The Leprechaun*. As he described this experience, in great detail, he became extremely animated. Brandon first described the stage make-up process, which included wrinkles, green face paint, and fake fingernails. He said it was a two- to three-hour play, and that his Dad came to watch it. 'It was a lot of work, but the audience loved it,' said Brandon with pride and much excitability. He stated that all of his lines rhymed and told how he had to memorize the script. He went on to describe it as a seemingly positive experience.

Brandon:	I've never told anyone this before.
Therapist:	What?
Brandon:	About being in that play.
Therapist:	Really?
Brandon:	I'd like to be a movie star one day...

COMMENTARY 1

A rapport had developed within the therapeutic relationship based on the patient's love of acting and recent experience in a leading role. Brandon was already looking forward to the drama sessions. 'The therapist must develop a warm, friendly relationship with the child, in which good rapport is established as soon as possible' (Axline 1947, p.75). Since

Brandon had a positive experience with acting in a theatrical production, the drama sessions should prove to be a familiar modality in which he can express himself.

Session #2: Jack and the Beanstalk

During the first dramatherapy session, Brandon selected the story of *Jack and the Beanstalk*. As the therapist told the story to Brandon, he listened very intently. He then selected the role of Jack to portray and asked that the therapist become the Giant. He stated that his favorite scene was when 'the beanstalk gets chopped down.' Brandon began the story during the scene where Jack shows the beans to the Mom:

Jack/Brandon:	Look, Mom! I've got beans…magic beans!!! [*He says with much excitement and fervor.*]
Mom/Therapist:	Where is Bessie? Oh, you sold her. Where is the money, Jack?
Jack:	No, there is no money, Mom. I've got BEANS…magic beans! Look!
Mom:	What? What have you done? Go to your room! No supper for you. Go. What were you thinking?
Jack:	[*Goes to his room, curls up on the office sofa and cries himself to sleep.*]

COMMENTARY 2

Brandon is extremely animated and very able to pretend, act and imagine. The first scene he selected to dramatize focused on Jack's being rejected by his Mother. It is Jack's need for maternal approval that is shattered by his Mother's anger. The therapist in the role of Mother berates Jack as in the original tale. Because Brandon is older than the other patients and more mature cognitively, the therapist does not feel a need to lessen the Mother's anger. Brandon is able to express much emotion during the dramatization and the therapist encourages this in-role. The tone of this scene changes drastically from Jack's sincere hope and excitability to his despair. Jack's trade of the cow for the magic beans is impractical, yet inherently good (Jones 1995). However, it is Mother's disappointment that leads to Jack's tears, which proves to be a loss of control.

As the fairy tale unfolded, Brandon continued in the role of Jack, and hid appropriately from the Giant, then proceeded to steal each of three objects: the hen that lays the golden eggs, the gold coins, and the golden harp. Each time he ran to Mother and was thrilled to tell her of the gold and riches. He held Mother's hands and literally jumped up and down. Then his favorite scene was enacted, when the Giant was coming down the beanstalk and Jack yelled to his Mother, 'Quick, an ax!' After he chopped down the beanstalk and the Giant had died, Brandon continued the story:

Jack: I better go make sure he is dead. What will we do with him now? Let's bury him, but how? [*Pantomimes burying the Giant.*] There, he's buried. No one will know...

COMMENTARY 3

Brandon, in the role of Jack, told Mother of the riches with much excitement and enthusiasm. This seemed to counter the earlier scene when Mother's disappointment had Jack in tears. This twist suggests approval- or attention-seeking behavior. His favorite scene was the most climactic of the story with Jack's saving the day, as the Giant fell to his death. He still required his Mother's help by calling to her for the ax. Brandon took the story further in his focus on the issue of death. Once Jack made sure that the Giant was dead, he proceeded to bury him, so that no one would know. This indicated that Brandon was beginning to explore the issue of death. It was the role of the hero, however, that was to become significant for Brandon.

According to Landy's taxonomy of roles (1993), the qualities of hero are defined as follows:

The hero journeys forth on a spiritual search that proves, in some way, to be transformational. This type is moral, inquisitive, and open to confronting the unknown. The classical tragic heroes are those who search for a meaning just beyond their grasp, willing to confront the hardships of the journey and to accept the tragic consequences that arise from uncovering certain elemental ambivalences of being. (Landy 1993, p.230)

The role of the hero, which was Brandon's preferred role, is clearly a young, healthy, and strong role to invoke. Brandon is young, but suffers poor health and is considered weak because of his chronic illness. The hero is wise and can outsmart the victimizer, so as not to become a victim himself.

The hero fights for what he wants. The qualities of the hero are those which Brandon would like to have in his everyday life. Because he isn't healthy or able to outwit his illness, he becomes angry and frustrated, which are emotions that are expressed through the role.

Brandon was to explore the role of the antagonist during the fifth, sixth, and seventh sessions, but then returned to the poor yet brave hero for the duration of the last three sessions. The hero is willing to face hardships in order to make discoveries that will shed light on his venture. Brandon needs to find a way to make sense of the illness that so adversely affects his everyday life. It is through the role of the hero that Brandon can fight hard and prove victorious.

As the hero, Brandon is able to take a journey facing unknown obstacles, only to become triumphant in the end. In the role of Jack, he risks his life time and time again, but the tragic consequences affect the Giant, who is the root of all evil in this tale. The Giant represents the very obstacles that Jack must not only face, but ultimately destroy. The Giant is the pivotal conflict within Jack himself, and is indicative of the fear and angst that Brandon struggles with in relation to his chronic illness. Brandon takes a risky journey and achieves resolution, although it may only be temporary. The function of the hero is 'to take a risky spiritual and psychological journey towards understanding and transformation' (Landy 1993, p.230). It is this spiritual and psychological journey upon which Brandon embarks, every time invoking the role of hero. It is a search for Brandon just as Jack searches for his own truth and resolution.

Session #3: The Gingerbread Man

It was during the next session that Brandon began to work with make-up. Make-up allows the patient to examine a role through the safety of distance. He had already selected the story of *The Gingerbread Man* during the previous session, and proceeded to select the title character. Brandon used brown make-up for his face, with purple cheeks and dark red lips. As he looked in the mirror he said, 'I look crazy.' He had applied the make-up with care and purpose.

When Brandon began the story, he curled up in a ball shape in the chair as the cookie dough. He became mixed, rolled, flattened, and cut into cookie shapes with the cookie cutter. Once he was baked and brought to life, the chase began. Brandon asked the therapist to be all the other roles in the story. When he ran, he actually ran very fast, yet in place, due to the confines of the small office space. As the story took off, with the cookie chase, Brandon added the energy for this action-oriented tale. He ran in place as fast as he could, calling, 'Run, run, as fast as you can, you can't catch me, I'm the Gingerbread Man.'

COMMENTARY 4

The near frantic pace of the running in place appeared to reflect Brandon's own frustration with his limitations regarding physical activities. Although the office space itself was small, and not conducive to actual running, it was the frenzied energy emitted by Brandon that suggested this link. The therapist, as narrator, was able to carefully control Brandon's physical exertion, by moving the story along. In this case, Brandon could act out his frustrations, through the monitoring of the narrator. According to both staff and his mother, Brandon could not participate fully in sports, such as football, and this proved to be very frustrating for him. His frustration often led to anger and to tears. According to Brandon's mother:

> *Physically he has a hard time. Today he was hospitalized, for example. He can't play football like he would want to. It's haphazard. He feels bad about it and he does love it [football]. Emotionally he gets angry. He is not able to play to his full potential. (Mrs J, personal communication, October 6 1997)*

Brandon's frustration and anger regarding his physical restrictions as they relate to his participation in sports, such as football, had developed into forms of denial. Brandon's primary nurse described Brandon's ability to make up stories. 'He denies it [his asthma] in some ways. Like it's never happened. He's very dramatic, making up stories about playing football. He tells about being on the team that won and all of the touchdowns he made...none of it is true' (DS, personal communication, September 23 1997).

By becoming the cookie in the story of The Gingerbread Man, *Brandon was given the opportunity to run for his life, if only through the drama itself. The gingerbread cookie was running as fast as it could while being chased by every character in the story. The cookie was fighting to maintain control or he would lose his life. He used sarcasm, taunting everyone he met to just try and catch him. The cookie was outsmarted by the fox, who was manipulative and victorious in the end. According to staff members at the partial hospitalization program, Brandon had an actual fear of loss of control, as was suggested by this story. The staff social worker stated, 'I know he doesn't like to lose control. That's very important to him. He likes to have control' (JM, personal communication, October 12, 1997). Brandon's primary nurse also explained that there was an indication of a fear of 'loss of control.' Brandon's frantic running during this session seemed to suggest this fear as it related, in part, to his physical restrictions, and his risk of asthma attack, which precluded any physical activity.*

Session #4: Hansel and Gretel

It was during the next session that Brandon selected what was to become his preferred story, *Hansel and Gretel*. After listening to the story, Brandon selected the role of Gretel. When asked, he stated that his favorite part of the story was 'all of it.' He decided upon make-up and proceeded to apply a flesh tone color to his dark skin. He then said that he wanted to be Hansel, too. Brandon selected two hats to differentiate the two roles he was about to play.

COMMENTARY 5

The therapist is aware that Brandon, who is African-American, purposely selected the Caucasian flesh tone make-up in transforming himself into Hansel and Gretel. He perceived the fairy tale heroes as being 'white,' which they are according to classic illustrations, and therefore altered his own appearance rather drastically in order to conform. He first selected the role of Gretel, who was the character responsible for outsmarting the Witch, and hence, the savior of the children's lives. Gretel was less directly threatened, as her brother was held captive, and because of her presence of mind and ability to think quickly, she prevented destruction. Brandon then decided to play both roles, which allowed for a certain security by becoming a team.

Stepmother/Therapist: So, Hansel and Gretel are going to the woods with us tomorrow and we're going to leave them. Well, we'll tell them to pick some berries or something but then we're going to leave them in the woods.

Gretel/Brandon: [*Gretel wakes up and hears the Stepmother's threats. She then wakes up Hansel.*] Did you hear that? Did you hear that?

Hansel/Brandon: [*Sleepily*] What?

Gretel:	[*Frantically*] They said they were going to leave us. They said they were going to leave us. And they're going to make us do everything and they're going to leave us in the woods right there and we ain't going to have no place...
Hansel:	[*Comforts Gretel*] It's OK, it's OK. I got a plan. I got a plan.
Gretel:	OK.

The next morning the Stepmother follows through on her threat as is described in the original tale. As the story unfolds, Hansel and Gretel find themselves abandoned in the woods.

Stepmother / Therapist:	[*To Father after sending Hansel and Gretel to find sticks and berries*] Now you, husband, time to go.
Father / Therapist:	I don't think I can do this [*leave his children in the woods*].
Stepmother:	Let's go. Let's just go.
Narrator / Therapist:	So the Stepmother and the Father went back into the house and they left little Hansel and little Gretel all alone in the woods.
Hansel / Brandon:	Huh?
Gretel / Brandon:	I told you.
Hansel:	Gretel?
Gretel:	[*Frantically*] Hansel, Hansel, I told you they would leave us. We turned around and they were gone. One minute they're here and one minute they're gone. What happened?
Hansel [*Calmly*]	Don't worry, don't worry. I left breadcrumbs. Breadcrumbs...breadcrumbs... I left breadcrumbs... [*notices they're gone*] the bird ate 'em! Catch that bird!
Bird / Therapist:	[*Using a bird puppet previously selected by Brandon*] Caw, caw, caw, caw.
Hansel:	Catch that bird!
Bird:	[*Bird flies away*] Caw, caw.
Hansel:	Darn [*sighs*]. What are we going to do now...

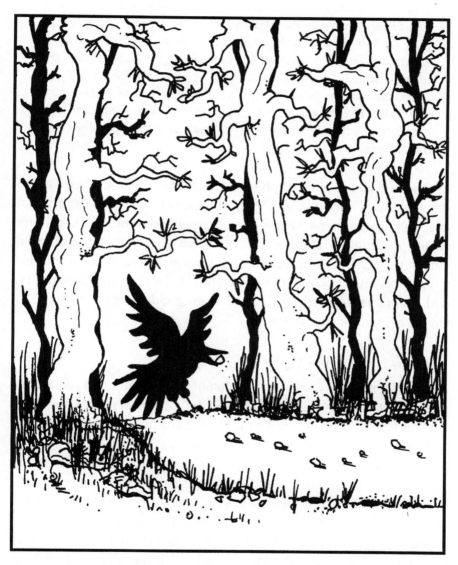

Figure 4.7 *The Raven stole the trail of crumbs, trapping the children in the darkness of the forest (illustration by Laurence Muleh 2001)*

COMMENTARY 6

The therapist portrays the roles of Stepmother and Father according to the tale as was told. It is important for the therapist to stay true to the story because of the tale's psychological significance and the dramatization's need for consistency. This structure allows Brandon the freedom to express himself through selected roles. Hansel and Gretel, one of the best known fairy tales of the Grimm brothers, deals with an oppressively hopeless situation. It is a story about abandonment. Not only do the children face abandonment, but desertion, solitude and separation (Mallet 1984). Fear of abandonment happens to be a potential effect of asthma (O'Dougherty and Brown 1990). Brandon explored the issue of abandonment and separation anxiety through a combination of the frantic helplessness of Gretel and the relative calm of Hansel.

As Brandon continued as both protagonists, he gave the witch's hat to the therapist for her role. The story unfolded according to the original tale. The heroes were successful and triumphant in the end. Brandon's acting was highly dramatic and animated. He was very motivated during the actual acting, yet remained somewhat cautious during his more direct interactions with the therapist. As he removed the make-up with the therapist's help, he literally said goodbye to Hansel and to Gretel, at least for that session.

Session #5: The Three Little Pigs

During the next session Brandon remained in his preferred role of the protagonist/hero, yet he also portrayed the antagonist for the first time. He selected the story of *The Three Little Pigs* and, after listening intently and with good eye contact, he stated decidedly that he wanted to be all four characters. When asked, he said that his favorite part was 'the brick part,' but that he really liked the whole story. Brandon asked the therapist to be the mom and then proceeded to select two masks to wear as the characters. A Wolf mask and a Pig mask were chosen.

The story unfolded according to the classic tale that was told at the beginning of the session. Brandon played the parts of all three Pigs. The Pigs were appropriately hungry as they ate their last breakfast at home and then they ventured into the world to make their way. The first two Pigs were naive and the oldest Pig was cautious and smart, just as the story goes. Once all the houses were built using pantomime, the Wolf entered and sneaked over to the house of straw.

Narrator/Therapist:	About that time, a mean and sneaky Wolf saw the house of straw and decided he was hungry for a Pig. So, he walked over to the house of straw and he knocked on the door.
Wolf/Brandon:	[*Knocks on the door.*]
Narrator:	And the little Pig inside said...
Straw Pig/Narrator:	Who is it?
Narrator:	And the mean, old, wicked Wolf said to the Pig...
Wolf:	Let me in, let me in.
Narrator:	And the littlest Pig of straw said...
Straw Pig:	Not by the hair of my chinny chin chin.
Narrator:	And the Wolf then said...
Wolf:	I'll huff and puff and blow your house down.
Narrator:	And the Wolf began to huff...
Wolf:	[*Takes deep breaths.*]
Narrator:	And puff as hard as he could, and then the straw was gone. It blew to smithereens and the Wolf started chasing the Pig and the Pig ran over...
Straw Pig:	[*Squeals*]
Narrator:	To his brother's house of sticks, ran inside and said...
Straw Pig:	The Wolf was chasing me and everything and he blew my house down.
Stick Pig:	It's OK. You're in a house of sticks. He won't be able to get you.

COMMENTARY 7

The therapist used descriptive narration between the dialogue in order to give Brandon time to change his masks for the roles of the Wolf and the Pigs. When Brandon huffed and puffed it was with such determination and effort that it appeared to be reflective of his own difficulty breathing. Mrazek (1993) describes an actual asthma attack:

*The muscles that line the airways tighten, constricting the route
through which air goes in and out. The lining of the bronchial tubes
swells and becomes inflamed, blocking the passage of air still further.
The mucus that ordinarily lubricates the airways becomes thick and
sticky and may actually plug them up. It becomes harder and harder to
breathe. (Mrazek 1993, p.196)*

*Yet, Brandon's intense huffing and puffing, as the Wolf, proved successful
as the first two houses were blown away.*

It was at the house of bricks that the oldest Pig said to his younger
brothers:

Brick Pig/Brandon: House of sticks? House of straw? What were you all
thinking? Well, you'll be safe in my house of bricks.

As the story continued, the Wolf knocked on the door, then proceeded
to huff and puff. When the house wouldn't budge, Brandon, as the
Wolf, roared with anger and frustration.

COMMENTARY 8

*Brandon's huffing and puffing elicited some actual wheezing. The
narrator consciously forwarded the story each time Brandon as the Wolf
huffed and puffed, in order to avoid any actual physical harm to Brandon.
The Wolf's anger and frustration in not being able to blow down the house
were reflective of Brandon's own frustration and anger relating to his
asthma and its consequential limitations. As previously cited, both the staff
and Brandon's mother had commented on his frustration and anger
regarding his illness. However, Brandon was not always able to verbalize
this concern.*

After the Wolf screamed from the bubbling pot, and the story ended,
Brandon was able to process some of his thoughts regarding this
session.

Therapist: Good job! Did you like that?

Brandon: It was a split personality [*laughs*].

Therapist: You had a split personality? Oh, because you had to
                 switch from one to another? Was it tough to switch the
                 masks like that?

Brandon:	Kinda.
Therapist:	Kinda, but it worked. You got to be four different people, three Pigs and a Wolf. Did you have a favorite of the four?
Brandon:	The smart Pig.
Therapist:	The smart Pig. He knew what was going on. The other two Pigs…
Brandon:	Yeah, they were lazy.
Therapist:	Now what was your favorite part?
Brandon:	When the Wolf tries to blow down the house. He gets tired.
Therapist:	Yeah, he got real tired and couldn't do it. Then what happens after he gets tired?
Brandon:	He tried to climb down the chimney, but he got mad.
Therapist:	He got real mad. 'Cause you got real mad, 'cause he couldn't blow down the house and he wanted those Pigs.
Brandon:	I like that story. [*Pause*] He mustn't have been walkin' fast.
Therapist:	He what?
Brandon:	He musn't have been walking too fast. He couldn't catch a Pig.
Therapist:	Oh, the Wolf? No, he couldn't have been too fast, could he? 'Cause he chased the first Pig and he chased the second, plus the Pigs were so scared, but he couldn't catch him.
Brandon:	But he was tired.
Therapist:	No, the Wolf couldn't be too fast 'cause he couldn't catch any of the Pigs.

COMMENTARY 9

The therapist used this informal questioning as a way to elicit information from Brandon regarding his character's motivations. This process may be more useful with older or more verbal patients. According to Brandon, the

Wolf couldn't blow down the house because he was tired. Also, the Wolf couldn't catch the Pigs because he was tired. This explanation was Brandon's own interpretation, as it was never described or suggested by the actual story. Brandon goes on to describe this tiredness resulting in the Wolf's anger. It is Brandon's tiredness from his asthma that resulted in his own anger.

The role of the Wolf is that of a beast. According to Landy's taxonomy of roles (1993), the beast is both physically and morally ugly. The beast of this story is physically strong, yet unable to blow down a house of bricks. The beast (Wolf) is not particularly intellectual and is motivated by his own untamed cravings. The beast is self-absorbed as the victimizer and is clearly anti-social. 'The function of the beast is to frighten and terrorize' (Landy 1993, p.176), as is exemplified by the Wolf's innate impulses. The Wolf depends on his breath, in order to survive. This directly related to Brandon's everyday life in terms of his everyday struggle to breathe.

As the sessions progressed, Brandon's acting continued to be highly dramatic, animated and motivated. He would change his voice, posture and attitude for each character that he assumed. During the interactions with the therapist, Brandon appeared more relaxed and less anxious. Brandon would, at times, select the story before the choice was given to him. Sometimes he would select the story during the end of the previous session. He would then select his role, before even hearing the story. Brandon knew exactly what he wanted to do. Brandon appeared eager.

Session #7: Jack and the Beanstalk

COMMENTARY 10

When Brandon explored the role of the antagonist, he only did so while also remaining in the role of the protagonist. This appeared to be a way in which Brandon could maintain control, which was an issue for him.

During the seventh session, Brandon selected the story of *Jack and the Beanstalk* again. He said he wanted to be everybody: 'As the external world, represented by roles, is internalized, one's inner world, represented by a system of roles, expands' (Landy 1993, p.35). By wanting to play all the roles, Brandon unconsciously is in need of expanding his inner role repertoire. This may be because of Brandon's need to surpass his own limitations. He then asked if the therapist would be the Giant's Wife and Jack's Mom. While selecting some costume accessories, Brandon told the therapist that he would be going back to his regular school after the first marking period, which had just started. He stated that he would be able to still come back and visit. Brandon's potential discharge from this day hospital program indicated that his health was improving.

As Brandon acted out this story, there was once again a focus on the moment when he, as Jack, was sent to bed without supper. After the Mother (therapist) discovered that Jack had traded the family cow for beans, she angrily sent Jack to bed.

Mom / Therapist:	Jack, is it you?
Jack / Brandon:	Yeah, Mommy, guess what I got?
Mom:	Where's the cow?
Jack:	I sold it.
Mom:	Good, where's the money?
Jack:	What money?
Mom:	No, no, no, let me see the money.
Jack:	There is no money, there's beans! Look, beans!
Mom:	What are these beans?
Jack:	They're magic beans. You know you can throw 'em and get a whole bunch of stuff and maybe get rich...
Mom:	Where's the money?
Jack:	There's no money. I sold it to an old man.
Mom:	For beans?
Jack:	Yeah.
Mom:	Beans?
Jack:	Yeah.
Mom:	Go to your room...
Jack:	But Mom...
Mom:	before I lose my temper. Go...

Jack:	Mom, but...
Mom:	Go.
Jack:	But...
Narrator:	Well, Mother was so mad, she threw the beans out of the window and sent Jack to bed without any supper. Jack was so upset...
Jack:	[*Cries from his room.*]

COMMENTARY 11

This particular scene was enacted with an array of emotions. The therapist was able to encourage Brandon's self-expression through the quick-paced and highly charged scene. Jack's initial enthusiasm rose to a crescendo, as the Mother became quickly angry. This, of course, led to Jack's upset. As Brandon lay crying on the office couch, he really appeared to be sad. Brandon reflected on the believability of this moment after the entire story was dramatized. This appeared to have been a cathartic moment for Brandon as was indicated by the intensity and sincerity of the emotion, as well as his recognition thereof. This was another example of the issue of abandonment or separation anxiety that was previously addressed through Brandon's dramatizations. A pattern regarding this issue was emerging.

As the story progressed, Brandon played the roles of both Jack and the Giant. Each time Jack took one of the Giant's treasures he climbed painstakingly down the beanstalk, only to have a confrontation with Mother. During his last escape the Giant followed.

Harp / Brandon:	Help, help, Giant! Giant!
Narrator / Therapist:	And the Giant woke up...
Giant / Brandon:	Uggh.
Narrator:	And started chasing Jack.
Harp:	Help, Giant, help!
Narrator:	Out of the castle, through the clouds, over to the beanstalk, and he ran and ran as fast as he could.
Harp:	Giant, help, master.
Narrator:	And the Giant was right behind him...

Jack:	Mom, Mom, get, get me…look at the harp, look at the harp. Get me the…get me the ax. Oh, my God. Look at the Giant!
Mom:	Oh, no, Jack, I told you.
Jack:	[*Groans as he cuts down the beanstalk.*]
Narrator:	And then the beanstalk went.
Jack:	[*Sound effect of falling beanstalk*] Thump.

Then Brandon paused from the drama for a moment to use the black make-up stick to create a 'blackened eye' for the role of the Giant. His last words as the dying Giant:

| Giant: | Kids these days [*dies and lies perfectly still*]. |

COMMENTARY 12

During this climactic scene, Brandon's characters became frantic and desperate. The role of the harp became shrill in its cries for help, while Jack became distraught among the frenzy. When asked what his favorite part of the story was, Brandon replied, 'When Jack runs up the stairs all those times.' By this he meant the beanstalk, but for Brandon the physical exertion required to act out this particular part of the story would equate to running upstairs. Brandon's serious asthma prevented him from any strenuous physical activity. It was Jack's running up and down the beanstalk which was Brandon's favorite part.

His favorite role continued to be Jack, the hero. The protagonist or hero continued to be Brandon's preferred role. It offered a certain success and triumph after struggling against adversities. During this session, Brandon became the threatening obstacle itself, the Giant:

They [Giants] personify the tremendous force of the unconscious, usually in its negative, destructive aspect. Views, discoveries and visions that are larger than life and can tear a man's psyche to pieces, may all take the form of Giants (i.e. experience which can't be formulated properly and may be very destructive). (Chetwynd 1982, p.169)

A pre-adolescent male who wants to play football and is told that he can't because of a serious medical condition may have difficulty in formulating this properly. Brandon touched on this force by becoming the Giant. When Brandon took on the role of the Giant, he was actually becoming his own fears, and therefore attempting to find a balance. By portraying both Jack and the Giant, Brandon was invoking counter-roles or opposing roles. This was one sign of successful treatment, as the patient is able to go to both sides of the struggle in order to find a resolution or a balance. Although the Giant died with a bit of humor, his death was very solemn and sincere. It was the role of the hero, however, that Brandon preferred. It was the journey that the hero took, that allowed for his own steps towards growth and understanding.

Session #8: Hansel and Gretel

Over the last few sessions, Brandon played only the protagonist roles. However, a noticeable change occurred in the hero's character. During the eighth session, Brandon returned to what was his preferred story of *Hansel and Gretel*. Again he selected both protagonists to portray. He applied stage make-up to his face using the flesh tone base color. Brandon selected two different hats to wear, one representing Hansel and the other for Gretel. As the story began, Gretel overheard the Stepmother's plans. She wakened her brother and told him what she had heard.

Gretel/Brandon:	Did you hear Stepmother?
Hansel/Brandon:	Stepmother? No.
Gretel:	Stepmother said she was going to leave us. She said that she was going to take us to the woods. That she was going to have us pick berries. Show us how to pick berries and they were going to leave us there.
Hansel:	Oh, you're lying.
Gretel:	No, I'm telling the truth.
Hansel:	OK. Wait until the morning, I've got a plan. Go to sleep. Go to sleep, go to sleep.
Narrator/Therapist:	So, with that, with Hansel's kind words Gretel fell into a deep sleep and they both slept for the rest of the evening, although they both tossed and turned. And the next morning Stepmother said:
Stepmother/Therapist:	Hansel! Hansel.
Hansel:	Leave me alone.
Stepmother:	Hansel and Gretel, get down here now.

Hansel:	Man.
Stepmother:	It's your Stepmother.
Hansel:	I don't care.
Stepmother:	Excuse me?
Hansel:	Nothing, Stepmother.
Stepmother:	Sit down for breakfast.
Hansel:	I don't want any breakfast.
Stepmother:	Well, all we've got is bread. Here's your bread.
Hansel:	I don't want any bread anymore.
Stepmother:	Are you talking to me?
Hansel:	I don't like bread. My mom didn't feed us bread.
Stepmother:	Well, I'm your mother now. Fine. No breakfast for you. Where's Gretel? Gretel! Gretel! Excuse me, here is your bread for breakfast. I think you're going to want this.
Gretel:	Um. I heard we're going somewhere today?
Stepmother:	Who told you that?
Gretel:	No one. It must have been a dream.
Stepmother:	Well. As a matter of fact, your father and I are going to be taking you out into the woods as soon as you've eaten your bread.
Gretel:	I don't want to go out into the woods.
Stepmother:	Excuse me?
Gretel:	I don't want to go out into the woods.
Stepmother:	Well, we're going and we're going now. Let's go.
Gretel:	I'm not done eating my bread...

COMMENTARY 13

Brandon's roles of both Hansel and Gretel had become defiant and argumentative. All of the protagonist's responses were negative and angry. This was a marked contrast to his early protagonist roles, which tended to be conforming. This particular role-playing was an indication of his need for control. Brandon was asserting himself in a way that was rebellious. He

didn't want to be told what to do. He was able to take on another perspec-
tive, and in doing so was also able to make that perspective his own. In this
instance Brandon was able to explore his own perspective by projecting it
onto the characters and then identifying with what he had created. This was
the first time that this pattern emerged and it was to develop further.

Once Hansel and Gretel found themselves abandoned in the woods, more anger emerged.

Gretel:	Hansel, Hansel.
Hansel:	What? I hate that old woman.
Gretel:	They left us.
Hansel:	You're lying.
Gretel:	They left us.
Hansel:	Duh!
Gretel:	What are we going to do?
Hansel:	I told you that I had a plan. You know that old bread that I had, that old, hard bread? That ugly stale bread.
Gretel:	Yeah, get on with it.
Hansel:	I left some breadcrumbs, OK. I left some breadcrumbs somewhere. OK. Where's the bread? I left some breadcrumbs somewhere. Where are the breadcrumbs? That bird.
Bird / Therapist:	Caw, caw.
Hansel:	Come here. Ahh!
Bird:	Caw, caw.
Hansel:	Darn it. I hate birds.
Narrator / Therapist:	And the Bird ate all the breadcrumbs and flew away.
Gretel:	Oh, what are we going to do?
Hansel:	I'm going to kill you, Bird. I'm going to kill you!

COMMENTARY 14

The issue of abandonment and separation anxiety presented a recurring
pattern in Brandon's dramatizations. His anger was expressed in this par-

ticular scene through his emotions and the dialogue. He described hating the Stepmother, and hating and wanting to kill the Bird. He even called the bread ugly. All of this heated dialogue was a result of being left alone in the woods.

As the story progressed, Hansel and Gretel devoured the house, outsmarted the Witch and then argued about their deeds. They fought over the riches and then confronted the Stepmother, until she apologized at their request. As the story ended, Brandon appeared very pleased with himself, as well as relaxed.

Brandon:	Aahh! [*Laughs*] He was a mean Hansel.
Therapist:	Yeah, he was, wasn't he?
Brandon:	He changed the whole story around.
Therapist:	Didn't he?
Brandon:	The witch said, 'You're as skinny as a stick,' and he said, 'So is your neck.' [*Laughs*]
Therapist:	He was feisty, wasn't he?
Brandon:	I liked that one.
Therapist:	Yeah, that was quite a twist.
Brandon:	Talk about changing the whole story around.
Therapist:	Yeah, Hansel took on a whole new self.
Brandon:	It was a calm one and a mean one.

Brandon went on to reiterate all the dialogue he had just improvised. He was very happy with all he had just expressed.

Brandon:	It was a whole different version of them two.
Therapist:	Now, how would you describe Hansel?
Brandon:	Hansel didn't like…he got tired of everybody always bossing him around. And he changed everything around. He changed everything that wasn't around…he changed everything…he just like, the bad version of Hansel.

174 PEDIATRIC DRAMATHERAPY

COMMENTARY 15

Brandon's feelings of a loss of control were combated by his defiance in the roles of the protagonist. Brandon's feelings of helplessness over his illness were indicated by the anger and manipulation expressed by these heroes. According to the clinical social worker at the hospital: 'Brandon... is a manipulator. He is the master manipulator. Sometimes he uses it [his asthma] when he doesn't want to do something' (JM, personal communication, September 23 1997). His portrayal of the role of the hero had taken on a transformation. Although Brandon described this new Hansel as being 'bad,' it is a role that Brandon needed to act out. In considering this role transition, it was 'the aim of treatment through the role method not to extinguish dysfunctional roles, like so many undesirable behaviors. Dysfunctional roles remain part of the system as foils and balances for the functional ones' (Landy 1993). Brandon now felt relaxed enough in the dramatherapy sessions to develop and express this 'mean' and manipulative character. It was a necessary exploration for Brandon.

Session #9: The Gingerbread Man

During the ninth session, Brandon returned to the role of the Gingerbread Man. The transformation that occurred for Hansel was to evolve into his role as the Cookie. Again, Brandon chose to use make-up. When applied to his face, it actually made him look like a cookie. He used white make-up around his eyes and called that the frosting. He used black make-up to create the gingerbread color for his face. He also made his lips red and described this as the licorice. He put on a black felt hat and described it as a cookie hat. Brandon's only statement, just as the story was about to begin, was, 'beware.' As the story unfolded, and Brandon as the Cookie came to life and began to run, his need for control was again apparent. This time the Cookie was insulting.

Narrator/Therapist: Then, all of a sudden, the Gingerbread Cookie came upon some farmers.

Farmer 1/Therapist: All right, give me that rake. Isn't it about time for lunch?

Farmer 2/Therapist: Hey, hey, Ed, look. Hey, you're a cookie!

Cookie/Brandon: And you're a human.

Farmer 2: I'm going to have you as a snack.

Cookie:	And you're very ugly.
Narrator:	And the farmers ran and ran, and they couldn't catch up with the Gingerbread Man as fast as they ran, and he was gone.

During the chase scenes, Brandon would run as fast as he could while in place. He would also let go a shrill laugh as he got away.

Narrator:	Then there was a horse.
Horse/Therapist:	*[Neighs and whinnies.]*
Cookie:	Hey, don't spit on me.
Horse:	I'm going to have you for dessert.
Cookie:	And you're very stinky! Nobody catches me… *[and another chase ensued]*.
Narrator:	Then along came a cow.
Cow/Therapist:	Mmmoooooo.
Cookie:	Quit making that stupid sound, it's getting on my nerves.
Cow:	I'm going to have you for dessert.
Cookie:	Milk, oh, milk yourself… *[and then the chase repeats]*.
All characters:	Cookie! We're going to have you for dessert!
Cookie:	I don't think so.

As is true to the original story, the Fox entered and offered to help the Cookie. With much hesitation the Cookie finally agreed to cross the river with the Fox. The Cookie climbed higher and higher on the Fox's back, but just as the Fox was ready to gobble up the Cookie, the Cookie was able to run to safety.

Cookie:	*[Running away]* You stupid old Fox! You thought you were going to get me.
Fox/Therapist:	I'll catch you yet, you cookie you!
Cookie:	I don't think so!

Narrator/Therapist: And the Gingerbread Man ran and ran and do you
know he got away from the Fox?

Narrator/Brandon: Then a little girl saw him and she played with him and
then she kept him as a toy.

Narrator/Therapist: And that's the story of the Gingerbread Man.

COMMENTARY 16

*Brandon was pleased with his rendition of this story. Although Brandon's
role was insulting and derogatory, it seemed necessary for his survival. The
'mean' quality of this role of the Cookie was similar to that of Hansel,
although more offensive. His abusive and hostile remarks seemed to
represent some actual feelings of hurt or helplessness that Brandon was experiencing. The sarcasm and hate that Brandon expressed through the role
of the hero were a defense mechanism to shield Brandon from his own pain,
both physical and emotional. Through Brandon's quick thinking, he was
able to outsmart the Fox and change the end of the story, much to his
advantage. He became a toy for a little girl, so that no one could ever
devour him.*

Session #10: Hansel and Gretel

During our last session, Brandon invited the therapist to come to his
school to see him do drama. He seemed sad that it was the last session.
He seemed ambivalent about his upcoming discharge. Brandon had
reported a headache earlier and the nurse had suggested he was 'the boy
who cried wolf.' This upset Brandon because he knew this to mean he
was being called a liar. He said he would discuss this with her later. He
proceeded to select his preferred story, that of *Hansel and Gretel*, and
stated that he wanted to be both the boy and the girl. He applied
make-up, once again his preferred projective technique. As he applied
the make-up to his face, he described the play he was once in, just as he
had detailed during our first session. Then he selected two hats to wear,
one for Hansel and one for Gretel.

COMMENTARY 17

*The quality of this session's story found Hansel to be more apathetic, and
resigned to their predicament. Gretel, on the other hand, cried when they
were left in the woods. The tone for this version of the story tended to be less*

spirited or driven than in previous sessions. There were often feelings of
ambivalence during a last session. Termination of a child's therapist can
appear as a form of rejection or abandonment to a child. Even if the reasons
are explained from the start. 'Closure is an opening up, another part of the
journey towards authentic existence that points toward the future, incorpo-
rates the past, and validates the present level of feeling' (Landy 1994,
p.120). It was Brandon's journey with a serious and restrictive illness that
lay before him. Through the dramatherapy, Brandon was able to explore
this path in trying to maintain some control over his situation.

During the processing of the final story, Brandon was able to reflect on
the difference in the protagonists from the previous session. He was able to
comment on the transformations that were evident in the roles of both
Hansel and Gretel.

Brandon:	I like the other, the old one better.
Therapist:	Which one?
Brandon:	The one I did with Hansel and Gretel before.
Therapist:	The last one?
Brandon:	Yeah. The one where Hansel was mean.
Therapist:	How was Hansel in this one?
Brandon:	He was mean and nice. He said, 'I could've stayed in here [the cage] all my life.' He said, 'You took kinda long.' Gretel was mean, too.
Therapist:	Yeah, she hadn't been mean before.
Brandon:	She said, 'You can hold that thought.'
Therapist:	Now what's your very favorite part of the story?
Brandon:	[*Thinking*] Mmmm.
Therapist:	Do you have a favorite moment?
Brandon:	The beginning.
Therapist:	At what point?
Brandon:	When they left 'em [*pause*]. Then the Bird ate the bread crumbs and Hansel started stomping on his hat. A whole bunch of people say I should be an actor. I wrote to Hollywood, again.

Therapist: Oh, yes?

Brandon: They haven't wrote me back again, yet.

Discussion

Brandon was initially presented as being appropriately cautious and somewhat reserved. He had a flat affect at first, and indicated some signs of depression. Brandon had good eye contact, but was minimally verbal during the first few sessions. He was seemingly tense, but there was a change in his behavior as the dramatherapy session progressed.

As the sessions evolved, Brandon became more at ease. His involvement in the dramatizations allowed him to become animated and expressive. This, in turn, gave Brandon an increase in energy and self-esteem. After each dramatization, Brandon became much brighter in affect, more verbally interactive, and overall, more relaxed. His participation in the role-playing was, from the start, a productive form of expression for Brandon. The role-playing proved to be a very compatible and non-threatening means of communication. Acting was natural for Brandon. He was extremely motivated from the start and, as the case indicated, was able to benefit greatly from this modality.

The Stress Measure, which was used as an observational symptom check list, was administered by the therapist after both the second and tenth session. Overall, the stress measure suggested that there was a reduction in Brandon's stress level (see Appendix A). The three major sources of stress in chronically ill children, which have been previously cited, were all issues that emerged within the dramatizations. Brandon's focus was on separation anxiety and feelings of abandonment. This issue was explored and emphasized as being his preferred part of several stories, particularly during his enactment of *Hansel and Gretel*. A pattern emerged regarding this issue, as it became a focal point of the dramatizations. The issue of separation anxiety was consistently adhered to from the beginning of the dramatherapy sessions to the last session.

Even more prominent for Brandon was the fear of loss of control. This issue was the catalyst for his characterizations during the last few sessions. As described during the case itself, Brandon's roles became demanding and controlling in an attempt to battle his own fear of losing control. Brandon's fight to maintain control was clearly reflected during the last few dramatherapy sessions. During the eighth session, for example, Brandon was in the roles of both Hansel and Gretel. Brandon was defiant and argumentative in his role-playing towards the Step-mother. He was indicating his struggle for control by this defiance. Brandon's freedom to express these conflicting emotions through the dramatherapy sessions had evolved over the ten weeks. There was an increase in Brandon's comfort level, whereas by the last sessions he was able to explore roles that suggested he was needing to be in control. As was previously cited, staff described Brandon as someone needing to be in control. With the recurring stress-related issues that were expressed, there was an indication of a reduction in stress for Brandon due to their eminence and his ability to vent them.

Interviews of parents and staff suggested that Brandon loved drama and was well motivated to attend each session. According to Brandon's primary nurse, 'He loves it [drama].' She went on to describe, 'Since he's had drama, his behavior is a little better. He thinks before he talks, rather than being inappropriate. His stress level has been reduced' (DS, personal communication, September 22 1997). According to Brandon's mother, 'He liked it [drama] very much.' When Brandon's mother was asked whether or not the dramatherapy sessions had any effect on her child's level of stress she responded, 'I mean for any child to act out or to perform will have less stress, and it will ease tension. It was a positive thing, not a negative. He wants to be an actor' (Mrs J, personal commu-nication, October 6 1997). The staff social worker stated, 'Knowing him I'm sure he loved it [drama]. He has a future in it. I think he's really quite an actor.' Regarding any changes in his behavior she stated, 'I think he's more aware now of some of the behavior things that he does' (JM, personal communication, September 16 1997). Overall, the staff and parent interviews suggested that Brandon not only had a love for acting, but also showed a reduction in stress due to his participation in ten dramatherapy sessions.

The CMAS-R was administered as both a pre- and post-test to Brandon. His pre-test score was 17, which is above average. His post-test score was 10, indicating a great reduction in stress (see Appendix A). Based on clinical observations, stress measures and instruments, interviews, and the issues presented in the case study itself, it appeared as though Brandon's stress level was reduced. The drama-therapy sessions were a productive intervention for Brandon, not only due to his motivation and passion for the art form, but because of their effectiveness in reducing his stress. The hospital was now planning to discharge Brandon at the end of the current marking period.

Six-Month Follow-Up

Brandon had improved physically and mentally during and immedi-ately following the dramatherapy treatment, as was described in the dis-cussion. Plans had been made for an upcoming discharge. Over the next six months, Brandon's medical condition worsened. Brandon had to be hospitalized. He was very sick over the school year, according to his primary nurse (DS, personal communication, March 23 1998). This past fall and winter seasons were considered to be very bad for asthma sufferers.

Behaviorally, Brandon had become very angry and moody regard-ing his chronic illness. Behavioral problems resulted and Brandon received an in-school suspension for the use of profanity and disruptive outbursts. Brandon had been attending a public school before his admission to the children's day hospital. He stated that he wanted to leave and go back to his own school. A possible discharge is being con-sidered for next September (DS, personal communication, March 23 1998). An extended dramatherapy intervention may have been helpful in not only reducing Brandon's stress but also in maintaining such initially positive results. Brandon is in need of a way to express continu-ally his anger and frustration. This incidence of recidivism may have been avoided if the dramatherapy intervention had been long term.

Transcript of selected session
Brandon: Selected Session #8 (9/9/97)
Brandon selects the roles of Hansel and Gretel.

> *Therapist:*   Then you can select what you need for Hansel and
> Gretel and you will be Hansel and Gretel.

	Now do you want me to be anybody in the story? Anybody else.
Brandon:	Everybody else.
Therapist:	Everybody else, OK. And do you know what your favorite part of the story is?
Brandon:	All.
Therapist:	The whole thing? All right, all of the story.
Brandon:	Which one is Gretel? The boy or the girl?
Therapist:	Gretel's the girl – Hansel's the boy.
Brandon:	It's got a lot of sprinkles on it [*refers to hat*]. Brush the sprinkles off.
Therapist:	I know there's sprinkles everywhere. So that'll be for Gretel. Oh great! And that'll be for Hansel. Oh good – good – good.
Brandon:	This is the second time I've used this hat.
Therapist:	I know – it's crinkly. It makes a crinkle sound. That's perfect.
Brandon:	Old-time hat.
Therapist:	It's an old-time story.
Brandon:	Old, dirty hat too because they're poor.
Therapist:	Oh yeah, they're poor, they're dirt poor.
Brandon:	[*Laughing*] She said they're dirt poor.
Therapist:	Is that right? Aren't they?
Brandon:	Uh-huh.
Therapist:	Because they have to sleep on like a little straw mat and everything else. So if there's any make-up, there's a mirror. It matches your shirt [*referring to hat*]. Every time you try on something it matches your shirt.
Brandon	[*Laughs*]
Therapist:	Didn't that happen last week?
Brandon:	Uh-huh. Hansel, Hansel and Gretel make-up.
Therapist:	If you want to use make-up you can. That's fine.

Brandon:	This is make-up?
Therapist:	Yes. That's the kind that you put on with your fingers. It all comes off with the make-up remover.
Brandon:	Oh that's cool.
Therapist:	Yeah, they're all stage make-up. Here are the make-ups.
Brandon:	Oh yeah, that what we used.
Therapist:	Did you use that for your play?
Brandon:	Yeah.
Therapist:	That's the good stuff.
Brandon:	What's this?
Therapist:	Sparkles – sparkle make-up.
Brandon:	That'd be too rich for her so I can't use that.
Therapist:	Yeah. Hansel and Gretel are very poor. So you're going to need poor colors. They can't have sparkles on them.
Brandon:	OK. I've got an idea. How long has this not been used?
Therapist:	We have some that a… Are we supposed to mix it with water? Do you need water?
Brandon:	I just put it on me.
Therapist:	Dip your finger in water and see if that makes it turn into make-up. [*Pause*] Does that make a difference?
Brandon:	Hold on.
Therapist:	[*Laughs*] Does that help?
Brandon:	I don't know.
Therapist:	Yeah, someone told me at the make-up place that if you add water to those that it makes it…
Brandon:	I'm just putting it on me – so I don't know.
Therapist:	Oh yeah. Well, look here – either I'll help you or you can put it on yourself. Either way is fine. Just so we remember to take it off before you go. Oh see, yeah, that works, doesn't it.
Brandon:	Em-heh. You put it all over my face. I can't do it 'cause that'll take too long.

Therapist:	You want this color?
Brandon:	Uh-huh, Hansel and Gretel, they're brother and sister. That water stays inside of it. Nice color, too. This is a poor color.
Therapist:	Doesn't it look like a poor color?
Brandon:	Em-heh.
Therapist:	I mean is this like dirt for them or is this their skin?
Brandon:	Skin. What should it be, dirt or skin?
Therapist:	Well, whatever you think. What do you think?
Brandon:	Well, we already have it on half of my face so it's skin.
Therapist:	OK. Let me see the other half of your face.
Brandon:	What are you doing, the sides of the face first?
Therapist:	Yeah.
Brandon:	That's the easiest part?
Therapist:	Right.
Brandon:	It'd be cool if it got all down here like the whole body.
Therapist:	Yeah, but that would take us two days to clean it off.
Brandon:	Yep. It took like an hour to put all the make-up on.
Therapist:	Oh, yeah. Now when did you tell me you're going back to school?
Brandon:	I'm not going back to that school that I had the fight. I'm going to another one.
Therapist:	Oh, like a middle school or something? [*Pause*] Are you going to do more plays when you go back?
Brandon:	I don't know.
Therapist:	Do you think?
Brandon:	Uh-huh.
Therapist:	You're quite good at plays.
Brandon:	I like acting. I wrote a letter to Hollywood. I'm waiting for the answer back.
Therapist:	Oh good.

Brandon: You know what for, don't you?

Therapist: No.

Brandon: Acting for real.

Therapist: Oh, really?

Brandon: People say that'll ruin your career.

Therapist: That what?

Brandon: That'll ruin your career.

Therapist: What will?

Brandon: Acting.

Therapist: Acting will ruin your career?

Brandon: Uh-huh.

Therapist: Acting for Hollywood?

Brandon: That's a nice color.

Therapist: Oh yeah, that's a great color.
                  Well, if you like acting, then you should always
                  remember to act. In school – in plays – anywhere.
                  Now, do I need to put some on your forehead or not –
                  with the hats?

Brandon: Yeah. It'll look better 'cause they show like...

Therapist: I'll just need to go up a little way. I don't want to get it
                  in your hair though.

Brandon: [*Laughs*]

Therapist: So you wrote a letter to Hollywood. What did you talk
                  about?

Brandon: Talking about I like most of the shows that they've
                  done. One person was Steven Spielberg.

Therapist: Get out of here!

Brandon: That's the first letter I wrote to was him. About his
                  cartoons and all that. Yeah, I like them. He wrote back
                  and said 'Thank You.' I talked to some people about
                  him. I was very, very happy [*Laughs*].

Therapist: Gosh, that's really big!

Brandon:	I didn't expect him to write me back, now.
Therapist:	No, that's cool.
Brandon:	Uh-huh. That's cool. I'll walk outside and everybody will say – like oh, you have two colors.
Therapist:	OK. Are you all ready to get started?
Brandon:	Yeah. Oh, where's the mirror?
Therapist:	Oh!
Brandon:	I forgot, I looked at the boy.
Therapist:	Did you look?
Brandon:	No, I only saw the girl.
Therapist:	Oh, yeah.
Brandon:	I don't like acting like a girl.
Therapist:	Oh, you said you don't.
Brandon:	I like acting as the girl, but I don't really act you know.
Therapist:	Oh, I know. But in Drama you can be either boys or girls, it doesn't matter.
Brandon:	I know.
Therapist:	All right.
Brandon:	But in real acting you gotta act as the boy.
Therapist:	Well sometimes they do both. It depends, you know. I did a play once with all girls, so they had to be the boys because it was a girls' school – 60 girls in eighth grade. They had to be the boys too.
Brandon:	[*Laughs*]
Therapist:	So you do both. OK, ready. Here we go. You ready? This is the story called *Hansel and Gretel*. A long, long time ago and very far away there lived a wicked old Stepmother and her Husband and they had a little boy and a little girl named Hansel and Gretel.
Stepmother/Therapist:	One night as Hansel and Gretel lay sleeping they overheard Stepmother say, 'No, that's it, tomorrow we're taking them to the woods. They can pick some berries, some sticks, you know I don't care what it is that they're

going to do but we're going to leave them in the woods! There's not a question, we're leaving them in the woods. No, no, there's no argument. We've got no food. We've got no money. What, do you want all four of us to starve?'

Husband/Therapist: And the husband said, 'Oh, dear. Oh, no I can't. I just can't.'

Stepmother/Therapist: Well I can and it's a done deal. Tomorrow Hansel and Gretel will become part of the forest, and that's final!

Narrator/Therapist: Hansel and Gretel had heard the Stepmother saying mean things about leaving them in the woods and they were very upset.

Gretel/Brandon: And that's when Gretel said, 'Hansel, Hansel, Hansel.'

Hansel/Brandon: Leave me alone.

Gretel/Brandon: Hansel, get up!

Hansel/Brandon: What, what? [*Laughs*] What, what, what? Oh, God.

Gretel/Brandon: Did you hear Stepmother?

Hansel/Brandon: Stepmother? No.

Gretel/Brandon: Stepmother said that she was going to leave us. She was going to take us to the woods. They're going to send us to pick berries and they're going to leave us there.

Hansel/Brandon: Oh, you're lying.

Gretel/Brandon: No, I'm telling the truth.

Hansel/Brandon: OK. We'll wait 'til the morning. I've got a plan. Go to sleep. Go to sleep.

Narrator/Therapist: With Hansel's kind words Gretel fell into a deep sleep and they both slept the rest of the evening. But they did toss and turn.

Stepmother/Therapist: And the next morning the Stepmother said, 'Hansel, Hansel!'

Hansel/Brandon: Leave me alone.

Stepmother/Therapist: Hansel and Gretel, get down here now!

Hansel/Brandon: Maaan!

Stepmother/Therapist: It's your stepmother.

Hansel/Brandon: Oh, I don't care!

Stepmother/Therapist: Excuse me?

Hansel/Brandon: [*Laughs*] Coming, Stepmother.

Stepmother/Therapist: I don't want any breakfast. Well, all we've got is bread. Here's your bread.

Hansel/Brandon: I don't want any bread any more!

Stepmother/Therapist: Are you talking to me?

Hansel/Brandon: Why bread? My mom didn't feed us bread.

Stepmother/Therapist: Uhhhh. Well I'm your mother now! Fine, no breakfast for you! Gretel – where's Gretel? Gretel.

Gretel/Brandon: [*Footsteps*] No, oh.

Stepmother/Therapist: Excuse me. Here's your bread for breakfast, I think you're going to want this.

Gretel/Brandon: I heard we were going somewhere today.

Stepmother/Therapist: Who told you that?

Gretel/Brandon: No one – it must have been a dream.

Stepmother/Therapist: Well, as a matter of fact, your father and I are taking you out into the woods as soon as you've eaten your bread.

Gretel/Brandon: I don't want to go out into the woods.

Stepmother/Therapist: Excuse me?

Gretel/Brandon: I said I don't want to go out into the woods.

Stepmother/Therapist: Well.

Gretel/Brandon: I don't like the woods.

Stepmother/Therapist: Well, we're going and we're going now. Let's go!

Gretel/Brandon: I'm not done eating my bread.

Stepmother/Therapist: Bring it with you!

Gretel/Brandon: I don't want to.

Narrator/Therapist: So Hansel and Gretel were very, very ornery and argumentative that day but the Stepmother and Father managed to get Hansel and Gretel out into the woods.

Stepmother / Therapist: And the Stepmother said, 'Pick some berries, don't be so lazy, good for nothing. Berries and sticks!'

Hansel / Brandon: You don't ever pick berries, why we gotta do it?

Stepmother / Therapist: Don't you dare speak to your stepmother that way! Berries and sticks.

Hansel / Brandon: Whatever.

Stepmother / Therapist: The Stepmother was furious and she said to the Father, 'Quick! They've gone looking for berries and sticks. Let's go, now's the time, now!'

Narrator / Therapist: By then, they were gone.

Gretel / Brandon: Hansel!

Hansel / Brandon: What?

Gretel / Brandon: I hate that old woman! They've left us.

Hansel / Brandon: You're lying!

Gretel / Brandon: They've left us. What are we going to do?

Hansel / Brandon: Well – told you I had a plan didn't I? You know that old, hard bread that I had, that old hard bread, that ugly, stale bread?

Gretel / Brandon: Yeah, get on with it!

Hansel / Brandon: I left some breadcrumbs, so we're OK. Where are the breadcrumbs? Caw-caw. The Bird! Caw-caw. I'm going to kill that Bird! Caw-caw. Come here! Darn it! I hate birds!

Narrator / Therapist: And the Bird ate all the breadcrumbs and flew away.

Hansel / Brandon: Oh, what are we going to do?

Narrator / Therapist: And Hansel and Gretel didn't know what to do. But just then the Bird returned as if to say –

Hansel / Brandon: Look at the Bird! Caw-caw. I'm going to kill you, Bird! Caw-caw. I'm going to kill you! Let's follow him!

Narrator / Therapist: And they followed the Bird as far as they could and then they saw what the Bird was showing them.

Hansel / Brandon: Oh my God! Ohhhhhh-wuuuuu! Look at that house, Gretel! I'm feeling quite homely now! Aren't you?

Gretel / Brandon: Yeah, I am. Let's go!

Narrator / Therapist: And they began to eat.

Hansel / Brandon: Gimme, I want that piece! Gimme! [*Chewing*]

Narrator / Therapist: Gingerbread, candy canes.

Hansel / Brandon: I want that piece too!

Narrator / Therapist: Sugarplums.

Gretel / Brandon: Ummmmm.

Narrator / Therapist: The best candy they had ever eaten in their entire lives. And then they heard…

Witch / Therapist: Nibble, nibble, like a mouse, who's nibbling at my house?

Hansel / Brandon: Did you hear that old, raggly sound?

Gretel / Brandon: Yeah, I heard it!

Narrator / Therapist: And they continued to eat.

Hansel / Brandon: Well – it's so good, I don't care what they say. [*Chewing*]

Narrator / Therapist: And then all of sudden out came a woman who said –

Witch / Therapist: Nibble, nibble, like a mouse, who's nibbling at my house!

Gretel / Brandon: Sorry, I didn't mean to eat at your…

Witch / Therapist: Oh, dear. Are you hungry? Come in. I'll fix you some lunch.

Gretel / Brandon: Wake up, Hansel, wake up!

Hansel / Brandon: Oh wo wo wohoooooo!

Witch / Therapist: Are you hungry, my dear? I won't hurt you. Come and sit down. I'll get you some nice lunch.

Brandon: [*Laughs*]

Witch / Therapist: Would you like a sandwich?

Hansel / Brandon: What kind?

Witch / Therapist: What kind would you like, my dearie?

Hansel / Brandon: Salami and banana and peanut butter.

Witch / Therapist: Right there.

Narrator/Therapist: So the old woman fixed them nice big lunches and drinks and sandwiches and everything delicious and they ate and ate to their delight – the most delicious lunch they had ever had.

Hansel/Brandon: Don't do that!

Gretel/Brandon: Shut up! Just pack it!

Witch/Therapist: And then the woman said, 'Well my little skinny! Come with me, my dearie.'

Hansel/Brandon: My little who? You called me skinny!

Witch/Therapist: I'm going to plump you right up with some more lunch. That's all I meant – some lunch.

Narrator/Therapist: And she pushed him into the cage and…

Hansel/Brandon: Oh, we'll get you, I swear!

Witch/Therapist: [*Laughing*]

Hansel/Brandon: Wait 'til I get out of here, I'm going to break you in half.

Witch/Therapist: Be quiet, my little skinny. Give me your arm, let me see if you're plump enough! Oh you're skinny as a stick!

Hansel/Brandon: So is your neck!

Witch/Therapist: Oh hush. Now my little girlie. Dearie. I'd like you to do some chores around the house.

Gretel/Brandon: No, my brother. Why did you do that to my brother?

Witch/Therapist: Because we're going to have a nice roasted dinner. [*Laughs*]

Gretel/Brandon: Why are you laughing? It's not funny.

Witch/Therapist: Come over here and make sure the oven works. We're going to cook a nice roast beef.

Gretel/Brandon: You little old witch.

Witch/Therapist: That's right, witch. Come on my dearie, here's the oven. Chop-chop. Chop-chop. Now lean inside the oven, my dear, and see if you can get it heated so we can make a nice roast beef.

Gretel/Brandon: Ummm, I don't know how to use this one.

Witch/Therapist: Well, think about it.

Gretel/Brandon: I don't know how to use it! I told you!

Witch/Therapist: Oh, you good for nothing!

Gretel/Brandon: Well, you do it then.

Narrator/Therapist: So the old witch leaned into the oven.

Witch/Therapist: Ahhhhh!

Narrator/Therapist: So the witch got slammed in the oven and Gretel ran over and opened the cage and let Hansel out.

Hansel/Brandon: That took you kind of long.

Gretel/Brandon: I could have let you stay in there.

Narrator/Therapist: And then.

Gretel/Brandon: You could have done it.

Hansel/Brandon: No, I wanted to do it. We're going to have witch.

Gretel/Brandon: I don't want any witch.

Hansel/Brandon: OK.

Narrator/Therapist: And then all the gingerbread cookies turned into children.

Children/Therapist: Hurray! You set us free. The witch had put a spell on us and made us into the gingerbread cookie house.

Hansel/Brandon: I didn't care.

Children/Therapist: Thank you so much. Thank you.

Hansel/Brandon: Oh, all right.

Narrator/Therapist: Then Hansel and Gretel ran to the house and grabbed all the golden riches.

Hansel/Brandon: Whooh! Get off there, I want that gold. Get off, Gretel.

Narrator/Therapist: They got the gold. They got the riches and they took everything home to the Stepmother and she said –

Stepmother/Therapist: What is that? Ohhh!

Hansel/Brandon: And you're not getting any of it.

Stepmother/Therapist: Gold, riches!

Narrator/Therapist: And then the Stepmother became quite nice when she realized they weren't poor.

Stepmother/Therapist: Oh, thank you, Hansel. Thank you, Gretel. We can live very happily ever after now.

Hansel/Brandon: You mean thank you for leaving us out in the woods?

Stepmother/Therapist: Oh! That was your father's idea. Because we didn't want you to be a...

Hansel/Brandon: I heard Gretel saying that you did it and Stepfather said that he didn't want to.

Stepmother/Therapist: Well, all that matters now is that we're rich, rich, rich, rich!

Gretel/Brandon: You mean Stepfather, Hansel and me are rich, rich, rich!

Hansel/Brandon: She said I'm sorry.

Stepmother/Therapist: I'm really sorry.

Hansel/Brandon: Well. Are you going to give us any more bread? Can we stay asleep as long as we want? With king-size beds? OK – and all my friends.

Stepmother/Therapist: Everybody. Let's celebrate.

Hansel/Brandon: All right. We're friends.

Narrator/Therapist: And with that Hansel and Gretel danced for joy because they were never, I say never, and I mean ever, poor again. And that's the story. [*Clapping*]

Brandon: He was a hero. He changed the whole story around. Didn't he?

Therapist: Didn't he. He was a tough cookie.

Brandon: The witch said, 'You're as skinny as a stick,' and he said, 'So is your neck.'

Therapist: He was feisty, wasn't he?
                    Oh wait, now let's take the make-up off.

Brandon: I liked that one.

Therapist: Yeah. That was a great twist to it.

Brandon: Talk about changing the whole story around.

Therapist: Yeah. Hansel took on a whole new...

Brandon:	There were the calm ones and mean ones. When the kid came out and said they were children, he said, 'Like I care.' Then they were arguing over the gold. Who's going to get the riches and all that. Well.
Therapist:	Hansel was feisty. Nobody was going to mess with him.
Brandon:	He said, 'I hate bread!' Then she said, 'Oh, what did you say?'
Therapist:	Right from the beginning, yeah. Right from the very beginning.
Brandon:	He woke up and said, 'Leave me alone.' He said, 'Oh, go to sleep.' He was calm to his sister until the money came.
Therapist:	He seemed nice to the sister like he really was going to help her. But the Stepmother – he had had just about enough of the Stepmother.
Brandon:	Uh-huh.
Therapist:	And the Witch!
Brandon:	He was mad at the Bird. He said I'm going to kill you, Bird. He was mad at that Bird.
Therapist:	Oh, that Bird. He got so mad when the Bird did that he didn't even realize that afterwards the Bird came over to try and help by showing him the house.
Brandon:	The best part was when he said he was skinny, the Witch said, 'so is your neck.'
Therapist:	Yeah, that made the Witch even madder. Although I don't even know if she heard it because she's so old.
Brandon:	Then, she tried to tell Gretel to light the stove and she said, 'I told you that I couldn't do it.'
Therapist:	Which part?
Brandon:	When she was lighting the stove. She said, 'I told you that I couldn't do it.' Then she kicked her in her bottom and she fell in.
Therapist:	[*Removing make-up*] This will loosen it and then all you do with the clean one is wipe. Now see if this one will just wipe it right off. Yes. See how that did that? So

what was it that he said, 'What took you so long?'
Because she threw him the key or something, didn't
she?

Brandon: And he didn't see it and he said, 'What took you so
long?' She said, 'I could have left you in there.' It was
like a whole switched version of them two.

Therapist: Yeah. I liked that. That was a great, great idea. Now
what did you say your favorite part of the whole story
was? Your favorite moment?

Brandon: When she said that, 'You're as skinny as a stick.' He said,
'Oh, so is your neck.' I switched the whole story
around. Oh my God, it's the first time I did that. You
can do what you want to?

Therapist: Oh yeah.

Brandon: I can do that? If I could do that, it would be funny.

Therapist: Describe Hansel. What was he like?

Brandon: He got tired of everybody always bossing him around
and he changed everything around. He changed everything. He's just the bad version of Hansel. Am I the first
person that ever did that?

Therapist: Yeah.

Brandon: I should do that in *Jack and the Beanstalk*. I should have
acted like hiding. I should talk back to him like I did.

Therapist: He was. He was talking back to the Stepmother and
making her mad.

Brandon: And at the end he got her.

Therapist: Yes, he did. He made her apologize. You know — and
make sure that it wasn't going to happen again.

Brandon: I need a little more of that cream.

Therapist: We're going to have to get you back.

Brandon: Yep.

Therapist: [*Continues to remove make-up*] Let me put on one more
layer of this. Right here — here — here. So there's a layer.
All right — then we'll just wipe that part off.

Brandon:	Can I have a paper towel?
Therapist:	Yeah. Oh wait – how about a tissue? Will tissues work?
Brandon:	Yeah.
Therapist:	We use lots of paper towels.
Brandon:	That's the best story I've done.
Therapist:	That was quite a story.
Brandon:	You were laughing sometimes while you were doing the story.
Therapist:	I know. You were laughing too.
Brandon:	[*Laugh*] I laughed to myself.
Therapist:	You laughed first, that's what happened. You admit that.
Brandon:	Uh-huh, I was laughing at myself.
Therapist:	That was really good though. And I'll be back again on Thursday.
Brandon:	The next story I know will really be good.
Therapist:	Oh, you already know?
Brandon:	*The Gingerbread Man.* But this time it's a different twist so he doesn't lie.
Therapist:	Oh?
Brandon:	He doesn't get eaten. I'll show you how. I'll show you. It's a whole different story.
Therapist:	[*Laugh*] All right. I'll have to admit that I like those twists. I have to admit it.
Brandon:	The best one, I think, if I do any other switches I'm still probably going to pick Hansel and Gretel.
Therapist:	Oh, if you do any other switches?
Brandon:	Em-heh.
Therapist:	That worked out really well because you said he was tired of getting told what to do.
Brandon:	I like the twist and you took off home with the gold.
Therapist:	Oh yeah. You did a great job. I'll have to admit.

Everything you can imagine is real.

Pablo Picasso

The Trickster

The following case study will be presented as a summary including a six-month follow-up and transcript.

Summary

Aaron is a 10-year-old boy with severe asthma. Aaron has aerosol treatments, oral medications, blood tests, and X-rays on a regular basis. His chronic illness proves to be frustrating for him at times. The difficulty in breathing can be painful.

The first story Aaron selected to enact was *The Three Little Pigs*. He chose the role of the Wolf. Aaron selected the part of the story when the Wolf was threatening to enter the houses. As Aaron huffed and puffed in order to blow down each house, he let out an actual gasping and wheezing sound that was clearly an indication of his severe medical condition. As he portrayed the Wolf, he used a scary, deep voice in combination with a latex wolf mask. Together, the effect was quite menacing. Aaron selected a role, that of the Wolf, which in this story is dependent upon its breathing in order to survive (the huffing and puffing down of each house). Because of his severe asthma, Aaron's survival is also reflected by his daily struggle to breathe.

Aaron was very attentive during the dramatherapy sessions, yet was minimally verbal. He appeared to have a lower comprehension level than would be considered average for his age. During the role-playing, Aaron paused to ask the therapist for some of the dialogue. Familiar phrases such as 'I'll huff and puff,' or 'nibble, nibble, like a mouse' were reiterated to Aaron, at his request.

Aaron portrayed the antagonist during every session. He began by exploring the Wolf from *The Three Little Pigs*, the Witch from *Hansel and Gretel*, and then the Giant from *Jack and the Beanstalk*. 'The antagonist strews obstacles in his [the protagonist's] path or actively seeks his destruction' (Thomas 1989). Yet, the antagonist, while threatening the

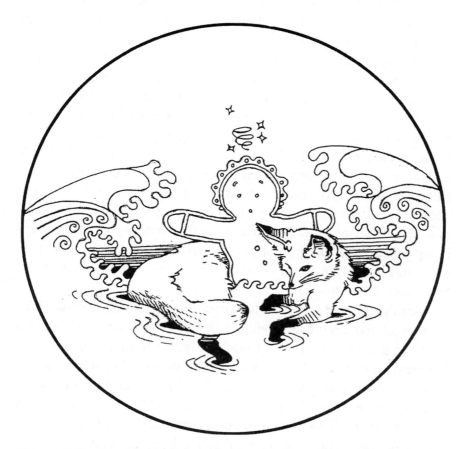

Figure 4.8 The sly and cunning Fox was the ultimate trickster (illustration by Laurence
  Muleh 2001)

child's very survival in a genuinely menacing way, always loses. One exception is in the case of the story of *The Gingerbread Man*, which was to become Aaron's signature story. Aaron's need to take on this type of role is indicative of his need to become the antipathetic force that he is otherwise compelled to face in his daily life as a victim. His primary nurse describes his most prominent issue as being a fear of loss of control (DS, personal communication, September 17 1997). By becoming the antagonist, the child may regain a feeling of control by terrorizing the helpless hero.

The Gingerbread Man is a cautionary tale. The cookie coming out of the oven is representative of birth. Yet developmentally, the cookie skips infancy, never taking the time to crawl or even walk. He is born and immediately runs, taking actual delight in being chased by animals and people alike. The young protagonist is trying to gain mastery as he runs haphazardly among all of the society that wants to devour him. As the cookie runs, having been chased, he gasps for air. According to Dr Salvatore Muleh, psychiatrist, asthma results in a fear of not getting enough air which can be referred to as 'air hunger' (SM, personal communication, January 11 2001). The breathless and gasping protagonist, being pursued by hungry antagonists, reflects this exact motif. In a sense, this hunger for air is a continual thread that is broken only in the final moments of this tale.

Aaron's preferred projective technique was the use of the mask. With the exception of his use of green face make-up to become the Witch for the third session, Aaron used a mask for every session. Masks have a 'powerful, transformational quality and in many cultures [they are] a means of communing with the spirit world, influencing the future, playing and releasing feeling' (Landy 1986, p.142). Aaron portrayed the role of the Wolf for the last six consecutive sessions while wearing a latex wolf mask. The Wolf is considered to be a universal beast.

> The typical representation of Mars, god of war, and death, in paintings, sculpture, tapestries, enamels, and miniatures, until the end of the fifteenth century, is a fierce-looking armed god of battle mounted on a chariot or cart. Almost invariably he is accompanied by a Wolf. (Rowland 1973, p.46)

The Wolf is, therefore, considered to symbolize death itself. There is never any sympathy for the Wolf. His punishment, as stated before, is always deserved.

A child with asthma may have a fear of dying by suffocation (O'Dougherty and Brown 1990). Interestingly enough, Aaron's preferred story was that of *The Gingerbread Man*, which he enacted for the last six consecutive sessions. The moment in the story which he repeatedly chose to act out was the scene in which the Gingerbread Man is forced to trust the Fox. Aaron referred to the Fox as a 'Wolf' for each session. Either the cookie was to climb further and further up the Wolf's back or he would drown, a form of suffocation. Inevitably, Aaron in the role of the Wolf would devour the cookie. As represented by the Wolf, 'the dark side of aspiration is devouring greed for substitutes that never quite satisfy' (Chetwynd 1982, p.155). Apparently the cookie satisfied the Wolf, in that Aaron repeated this exact scene over and over again, each week.

Narrator/Therapist: So, the cookie said to the cow:

Gingerbread Man/Therapist: Run, run, as fast as you can. You can't catch me, I'm the Gingerbread Man.

Narrator: And the cookie ran and ran and ran as fast as the cookie could. The cookie, all of a sudden, ran over to a river.

Gingerbread Man: Uh, oh [*and then the cookie thought...*]. How am I going to cross the river, because I'm a cookie and I might dissolve?

Narrator: Then the cookie looked back and there they were. There was the Farmer, the Farmer's Wife, the Farmers from the field, the horse, and the cow. They were all yelling at the cookie. They were saying:

Gang/Therapist: Cookie, cookie! We're going to have you for dessert! Cookie!

Gingerbread Man: Run, run, as fast as you can, because you can't catch me, I'm a Gingerbread Man.

Narrator: But the Gingerbread Man didn't know how to cross the river, so he said:

Gingerbread Man: Uh, oh. What am I going to do?

Narrator:	And just then out came a Wolf. And the Wolf said:
Wolf/Aaron:	I'll take you across.
Gingerbread Man:	Uhhh…
Wolf:	I won't eat you.
Gingerbread Man:	Uh, you won't?
Wolf:	No.
Gingerbread Man:	Do you promise?
Wolf:	Yup.
Gingerbread Man:	Uh, I don't think I'd better. I don't think I'd better.
Narrator:	But then the group of people kept calling and getting closer and closer.
Gang:	Cookie. Come back here, cookie!
Narrator:	And the cookie said:
Gingerbread Man:	OK, OK. I'll do it.
Wolf:	Jump on my back.
Gingerbread Man:	All right.
Narrator:	So the cookie jumped on top of the Wolf's back and started to go up the river.
Gingerbread Man:	Hey, wait…my feet are getting wet.
Wolf:	Jump on my shoulders.
Gingerbread Man:	Now that's much better. Thank you, Wolf. That's a great idea. Run, run, as fast as you can. You can't catch me I'm a Gingerbread Man. Ha ha ha! Hey, my feet are getting wet!
Wolf:	Jump on my head.
Gingerbread Man:	Run, run as fast as you can. You can't catch me, I'm the Gingerbread Man. Hey, my feet are getting wet.
Wolf:	Jump on my nose.
Narrator:	So, the cookie jumped up on top of the top of the Wolf's nose and then all of a sudden the Wolf went…

| *Wolf:* | [*Gulp*] Mmmmm. |
| *Narrator:* | And the cookie was gone. And that's the story of *The Gingerbread Man.* |

The role of the Fox is one of deceit. The function of the Fox is to trick. His motivations are self-serving. The qualities of this role are cunning and wit. The Fox in *The Gingerbread Man* is the only antagonistic character that is victorious in the end. Every other Witch, Wolf, or Giant from the other fairy tales is defeated by the protagonists. The Fox is like the role of the trickster defined in Landy's taxonomy of roles in terms of his mischievous and amoral qualities (Landy 1993). The Fox is presentational in style, due to his much overdistanced and emotionless manner.

The significance of the trickster is explored in *Storymaking in Education and Therapy* (Gersie and King 1990, p.191). The trickster is one of seven themes reflective of universal tales and myths, which can define human experience:

> Trickster fearlessly treads where most are reluctant to go; without love and without hate, acting and dreaming the wildest dreams in order to realize them all. There is no choosing. (p.193) The trickster promises nothing, or if he does, it is meaningless as in the case of the fox in *The Gingerbread Man*. He is simply not to be trusted. One can not control, understand or appreciate the trickster for it is…the one who dwells within us (that) is the one we encounter without in a time of danger. (Gersie and King 1990, p.191)

Aaron's role of the Fox was not playful, but serious in its challenge to succeed. This seriousness is further indicated by the repetitiveness of Aaron's role selection. If the dramatherapy sessions had continued, Aaron may have been able to explore alternative counter-roles in an attempt to achieve a balance. However, due to the significance of this role for Aaron, he needed to act it through repeatedly. The Fox, which Aaron referred to as the Wolf, symbolizes death (Chetwynd 1982), which is unfortunately a part of Aaron's everyday reality.

Aaron enacted this same scene each week. Each time he wore the Wolf mask, except for one day, when he came to drama wearing a medical mask that covered his nose and mouth. Aaron wore the medical mask in order to avoid the transmission of bacteria due to a cold sore he

had developed. Aaron used his medical mask as his Wolf mask that day.
As the sessions unfolded, Aaron remained minimally verbal. He was
able to express himself by dramatizing the same scene from *The Gingerbread Man*, repetitively. Yet his interactions with the therapist, when not
in role, continued to be mostly 'uh-huhs' and nodding to respond. He
rarely initiated a conversation, other than through the dialogue of his
favorite story.

Towards the end of the therapy sessions there was a two-week
interval when dramatherapy wasn't held due to the partial hospital's
summer schedule. During this time, Aaron became sick.

Therapist:	I'm sorry that I haven't seen you in a while, because last week everyone had vacation and the week before was a teacher's in-service. So, I haven't seen you in a couple weeks, but I am back and we still have a few sessions together for drama. Now, how have you been?
Aaron:	Good.
Therapist:	I understand that you were in the hospital?
Aaron:	Uh huh.
Therapist:	Really? When was that?
Aaron:	Monday.
Therapist:	For the day?
Aaron:	No.
Therapist:	For more than a day?
Aaron:	Yup.
Therapist:	How many days?
Aaron:	Three.
Therapist:	What was wrong?
Aaron:	Asthma attack.
Therapist:	Oh, really? Were you here in this hospital?
Aaron:	Uh uh.
Therapist:	Somewhere else?
Aaron:	Uh huh.

Therapist:	Where did you go?
Aaron:	[*Names hospital.*]
Therapist:	How was that?
Aaron:	Good.
Therapist:	Did they take care of you?
Aaron:	Yep.
Therapist:	Good! Oh, so you must have had an asthma attack on Labor Day, Monday? Was that scary [*pause*] or no?
Aaron:	No...

Often children with chronic or life-threatening illnesses do not want to talk about it. Aaron is representative of this norm. Having spoken with Aaron's primary nurse from the pediatric hospital where he had been hospitalized as an inpatient, it was learned that he had been 'very near death on more than one occasion' (KW, personal communication, September 16 1998). This explained why he repeatedly acted out the role of the Wolf, which symbolizes death. It was also revealed that Aaron has a hearing impediment. This explained his seeming indifference at times, which was indicated by his minimal verbalizations. Apparently, Aaron had trouble hearing, but had not mentioned it. The staff of the partial hospital program never mentioned this.

Aaron's social worker said that there were marked changes since Aaron completed dramatherapy:

> He doesn't do that silly laughing any more. He used to laugh all the time. It was a nervous laugh, and very inappropriate. He was very talkative in a disruptive way. He was very loud. He hasn't done it since the end of the summer. It was uncontrollable laughter. (JM, personal communication, September 13 1998)

According to several staff members, Aaron came from a chaotic and troubled home. Aaron's negative behaviors had improved since the summer, and since he had dramatherapy. 'He used to scream and yell, but now he's doing well in school. His negative behaviors have improved. His stress had decreased a little, but his asthma is still bad' (CJ, personal communication, September 10 1998). She went on to describe that he does have a fear of a loss of control.

Aaron's dramatherapy sessions were primarily focused on the same climactic scene from the same story, that being *The Gingerbread Man*. Almost every week Aaron became the Wolf and lied to the cookie, in order to devour him. The Wolf was clever and witty, more so than any other character in the story, and therefore outwitted the cookie. The Wolf is the only antagonist within the five fairy tales that had been previously selected that survived. This scene represents fear of bodily harm or death and a fear of loss of control. The Wolf proves to be very calculating in maintaining his control and all-knowing, thus the Gingerbread Man gets consumed. The Wolf eats the cookie for his own survival. Aaron's repetition of this particular dramatization indicates a need to explore this conflict.

The Children's Manifest Anxiety Scale – Revised (CMAS-R) was administered as both a pre- and post-test. Aaron's pre-test score was 14, which is just above the mean score of 13.84. Aaron's post-test score was 4. This indicates a great reduction in stress/anxiety. Therefore, according to the CMAS-R results, Aaron's stress was greatly reduced.

Based on the stress-related issues expressed through the dramatizations, interviews and psychological instruments administered, it appeared as though Aaron's stress level decreased after his participation in the dramatherapy study. Although his role enactment became singularly focused, it was clearly necessary for Aaron to explore this specific climactic moment of the same story, over and over again. The power of becoming the role of the Wolf (representing death) was very significant for Aaron, having faced his own mortality on more than one occasion.

Six-Month Follow-Up

Aaron's medical condition had improved somewhat over the six months, since the dramatherapy treatment. Aaron has had two hospitalizations since September of 1997. He is being considered for discharge by the fall of 1998. Although his health has improved, Aaron had recently indicated some symptoms of stress because some of the other patients in the program had been teasing him. According to Aaron's primary nurse, Aaron was 'not fitting in' (DS, personal communication, March 23 1998). Some of the other patients, more particularly the adolescents, were referring to Aaron as a girl because of his longer hairstyle.

Six months ago Aaron was able to ignore the teasing, but apparently over the past few months the teasing had become upsetting for him. This appears to be a stress-related issue that has been instigated and re-inforced by peer pressure. In spite of this nominal setback, Aaron's health has shown improvement.

Transcript of selected session

Aaron: Selected Session #8 (9/9/97)

Therapist:	Now, for today as always…oh, we need to do the questionnaire today…we'll still have drama again this week. But, I'm going to name for you five stories. The same five stories that we've always had. And you can pick any story…
Aaron:	*The Gingerbread Man.*
Therapist:	You know already?
Aaron:	[*Nods*]
Therapist:	Well then, for today we will do *The Gingerbread Man.* If we do *The Gingerbread Man* who would you like to be?
Aaron:	The Wolf.
Therapist:	And who would you like for me to be?
Aaron:	[*Shrugs*]
Therapist:	Doesn't matter?
Aaron:	Uh-uh.
Therapist:	All right. Um. Which part of the story should we do? The whole story or just the part that the Wolf's in?
Aaron:	The part with the Wolf.
Therapist:	Do you want me to tell you the whole story or do you remember it?
Aaron:	I remember it.
Therapist:	OK. If you would like to use anything from inside the…
Aaron:	[*Nods no*]
Therapist:	Nothing today?

Aaron:	Uh-uh [*no*].
Therapist:	You have on your own mask today? [*Referring to the medical mask that he is wearing in order to avoid the transmission of disease.*]
Aaron:	Uh huh [*yes*].
Therapist:	Is that because you have a cold or something?
Aaron:	Uh-uh [*no*].
Therapist:	Why do you have to wear...
Aaron:	Cold sore [*inaudible*].
Therapist:	Huh?
Aaron:	Cold sore.
Therapist:	Oh, a cold sore. So you have to wear that?
Aaron:	Uh huh [*yes*].
Therapist:	Well, it seems almost like a mask? Doesn't it?
Aaron:	Uh huh.
Therapist:	Do you want that to be your Wolf mask?
Aaron:	OK.
Therapist:	OK. All right, do you want me to be the cookie? [*Pause*] Did you want to be the cookie?
Aaron:	Uh-uh [*no*].
Therapist:	No, you're going to be the Wolf.
Aaron:	Uh huh.
Therapist:	I can be the cookie. Where should we start the story from?
Aaron:	When the Wolf comes in.
Therapist:	Oh, yes. Right when the Wolf comes in. Where does he come from? [*Pause*] Do you think that when he comes in and sees the cookie that he knows what he wants?
Aaron:	Uh huh.
Therapist:	All right. We're going to act out our story. We'll start right there at that one point. We won't do the whole thing. We'll start right there. Do we need anything?

Aaron:	[*Nods no.*]
Therapist:	You don't need anything from the bag today?
Aaron:	Uh-uh.
Therapist:	You're going to use that as the mask?
Aaron:	Uh huh.
Therapist:	All right. That's good. And, umm, I'm the cookie. Now, somebody was just chasing me. Now who was it? [*Pause*] Oh, the people and the animals were chasing me.
Aaron:	Uh huh.
Therapist:	You ready?
Narrator / Therapist:	And the cookie said:
Cookie:	Run, run, as fast as you can, you can't catch me, I'm the Gingerbread Man!
Narrator / Therapist:	And the cookie ran as fast as he could. As fast as a cookie could go. Away from the horse, away from the cow, away from the farmer, the farmer's wife and from the people out in the field. The cookie ran and ran and ran. And nobody, I mean nobody, was going to get that cookie. And then the cookie said:
Cookie:	Oh! Uh, oh? There's a river. [*Gulp*] How am I going to get across that river? I'm just a cookie and if I dare to put my foot in the river I would surely melt. Oh, they're coming, they're coming after me!
Narrator:	And everybody was saying
Gang:	Hey you – cookie! We're going to have you for dessert. Cookie!
Cookie:	And the cookie said, 'Run, run, as fast as you can, you can't catch me a...uh, oh. What am I going to do?'
Narrator:	And just then the cookie looked over and saw a Wolf and the cookie said...
Cookie:	Oh, who are you?
Wolf / Aaron:	The Wolf.

Cookie: Oh, look. You're not having me for dessert. [*Pause*] Do you think you could help me?

Wolf: I'll take you across.

Cookie: You'll take me across the river? No way.

Wolf: Yes.

Cookie: No, because you'll gobble me up.

Wolf: No, I won't.

Cookie: Promise?

Wolf: Yeah.

Cookie: Honest?

Wolf: Yup.

Narrator: The cookie didn't know what to do, but he felt like he had no choice and so the cookie said…

Cookie: OK. What'll I do?

Wolf: Jump on my back.

Narrator: So, the cookie jumped up on the Wolf's back and the Wolf began to go across the river. [*Therapist places her hands on the Wolf's back to represent this.*]

Cookie: Oh, thank you so much Mr Wolf. Oh, you're really saving my very life. Do you know that those people over there wanted to have me for lunch? Run, run, as fast as you can, you can't catch me, I'm a Gingerbread Man, ha ha. Hey, my feet are getting wet!

Wolf: Jump on my shoulders. [*Aaron proceeds to circle around the office as if swimming across the water.*]

Cookie: There [*moves hands to shoulders*] that's much better. Run, run, as fast as you can and you can't catch me, I'm the Gingerbread Man. Hey, the water is getting higher. My feet are getting wet!

Wolf: Jump on my head.

Narrator: So, the cookie jumps on his head [*places her hands on his head*].

Cookie:	That's better. That's much, much, much better. Uh-oh, my feet are getting wet!
Wolf:	Jump on my nose.
Cookie:	Oh, all right.
Narrator:	And then all of a sudden the wolf went...
Wolf:	[*Gulp*] Mmmmm.
Narrator:	And the cookie was gone and that's the story of *The Gingerbread Man.*
Therapist:	Good job. When we went around and around like that, did that make you dizzy?
Aaron:	[*Nods no.*]
Therapist:	That's because you were the Wolf. Yes, and the Wolf ate the cookie. The cookie was no more. Good story. Now what's your favorite part of the story?
Aaron:	[*Inaudible*]
Therapist:	Hmm?
Aaron:	All of it.
Therapist:	The whole story? [*Pause*] Well, that worked, because that's almost like a mask you were wearing. [*Pause*] So, you could just wear this mask instead. [*Pause*] OK. Only with this mask, I can see your eyes.
Aaron:	Uh huh.
Therapist:	The other mask, I could barely see a bit of your eyes, from behind the Wolf. Very good. Now, I have to ask you some questions from the questionnaire. Remember when we first did this at the beginning of the summer? [*Pause*]. It's yes and no answers. I'll say the sentence and then you say yes or no. So, we can go ahead and get this done and then we'll meet again on Thursday. OK, you ready?
Aaron:	Uh huh [*proceeds to take C.M.A.S.-R. post-test, giving yes and no answers*]

Therapist:	[*After it's done*] Thank you for that. Is your favorite story *The Gingerbread Man*?
Aaron:	Uh huh.
Therapist:	And is your favorite part with the Wolf? [*He's already mentioned this in previous sessions.*]
Aaron:	Uh huh.
Therapist:	And what do you like best about the Wolf?
Aaron:	He's mean.
Therapist:	He is mean, isn't he.
Therapist:	He's so mean. He stands there and says, 'No, I won't eat you,' then says, 'Jump on my back.' And the next thing you know... [*Pause*] All right, I'll plan to see you on Thursday.

One does not become enlightened imagining figures of light, but by making the darkness conscious.

C.G. Jung

The Bubbling Pot

The following case study will also be presented as a summary and includes a six-month follow-up and transcript.

Summary

Glen is a 7-year-old boy with severe asthma, a condition he has suffered from since birth. His extensive daily medications include prednisone; the steroids he takes cause his face to be very full and puffy. Among the noticeable side effects of his medication, Glen has had immense weight gains, having actually added 40 pounds to his 60-pound body in the recent past. Glen also has extensive food allergies, necessitating a very restrictive diet. For example, he must drink baby formula instead of milk and cannot have ice cream. Due to the severity of Glen's condition, he has been hospitalized several times. Overall, he was described as a well-adjusted boy with a supportive family.

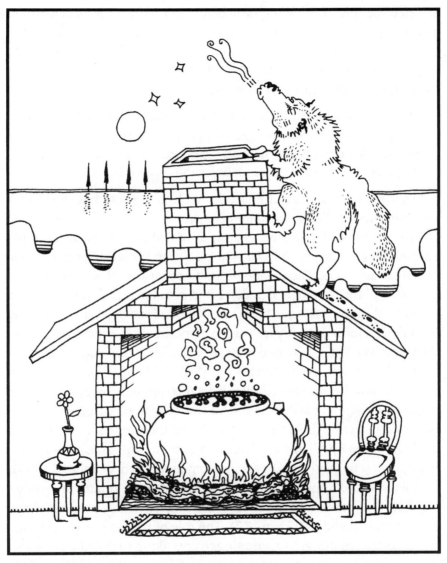

Figure 4.9 As the Wolf climbed up the roof to the chimney, he let out a howl into the darkness of the night (illustration by Laurence Muleh 2001)

Glen was an attentive and motivated boy. The fairy tale he selected during the first session, *The Three Little Pigs*, became his preferred story. He described this as being his favorite story. Glen was animated and eager during the initial session, appearing quite verbal. Although he selected the role of the Wolf, he actually proceeded to act out the roles of the Pigs as well. Playing the Wolf, he donned a mask, but as the Pigs he sported a crown. With his puffy cheeks from the prednisone and growth retardation due to the steroids, he actually resembled a piglet. According to his clinical social worker:

> Have you ever seen kids on prednisone? [*Pause for response.*] Well, he was grotesque. He now weighs 60 pounds and he was almost 100 pounds. 40 pounds on that little creature. He looked like a big chipmunk. (JM, personal communication, September 18 1997)

When Glen huffed and puffed as the Wolf, it appeared as though his breathing was difficult and somewhat labored.

During the second session, Glen applied make-up to become the 'old Farmer' in *The Gingerbread Man*. He used gray for wrinkles and added brown as age spots. Glen made himself appear old. It was during this session, and the last, that Glen described how his grandmother used to read him these same stories. It appeared to be a fond memory. According the Glen's mother, 'Last year his grandmother and great-grandfather died and my sister had two miscarriages. That was rough' (Mrs D, personal communication, October 6 1997). The loss of his grandparents may have been reflected by the detailed application of the old age make-up. When he played the role of the Farmer, he gasped heavily as he toiled in the field. As the Farmer chased the cookie, he panted and could not keep up. Glen's medical condition precludes his participation in physical activities (Mrs D, personal communication, October 6 1997).

Glen's exploration of the role of the elder is found in Landy's taxonomy of roles. The elder is 'wise, philosophical, prophetic, and sympathetic' (Landy 1993, p.172). The role of the elder is realistic and representational in style, functioning to pass along the wisdom of experience to the younger generations (1993). Glen's invoking of the role of elders may have been related to the recent death of his grandmother and great-grandfather. The role of the elder is not as final or bleak as the role of death, which was explored in several other cases. The role of elder seemed to offer some sense of security to Glen's dramatizations.

As the sessions unfolded, a pattern emerged as Glen portrayed both the protagonist and the antagonist. This was to occur during almost every session. Glen needed to play opposing forces: the weak battling the strong, the strong against the weak. When acting out *Jack and the Beanstalk*, Glen stated, 'I'm the little boy and the big Giant.' This seemed to give Glen a sense of control. He continued by narrating the story, in addition to playing the roles of the protagonist and the antagonist. He continued to be animated and expressive.

During the fifth session, Glen selected the story of *Little Red Riding Hood*. After listening intently while the therapist told the story, Glen was asked what character he would like to be. He settled on the roles of Little Red Riding Hood and the Tiger (Wolf). As he looked through the drama bag, he found a cap for Grandmother, a wolf mask for the Tiger/Wolf and a sailor hat for the Huntsman. He described the Huntsman as a retired Sailorman, once again creating an elderly character. Glen found a hood and a cape for Little Red and some puppets to portray the woodland animals. He told the therapist to be the Mother and he assumed all other roles.

Glen acted as Little Red, the Wolf, Grandmother, and the Huntsman. As the story progressed, Glen enacted all these roles in a manner true to the original story. As the story ended, with the retired Sailorman/ Huntsman rescuing Little Red and Grandmother, the scene shifted to Mother's house. Mother was worried about Little Red, and for good reason.

Mother/Therapist: Little Red has been gone for so long now that I'm really beginning to worry.

Glen: Pretend that you come out to look for me.

Mother: I'm going to go out and look for Little Red. I told her not to talk to strangers and to stay on the path. She should've been home by now. I have a very bad feeling about this.

Narrator/Therapist: So Mother got her purse and hat and went out looking for Little Red.

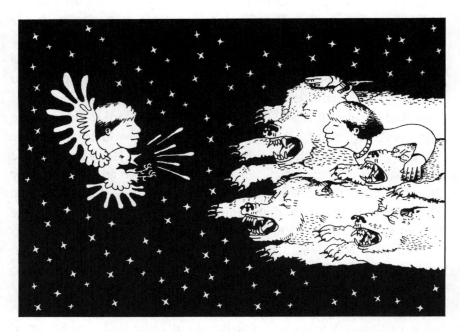

*Figure 4.10 In a clash of emotions, Glen fought to overcome his innermost fears
(illustration by Laurence Muleh 2001)*

Mother:	Little Red, Little Red! I guess I'll have to make my way all the way to Grandmother's house. Oh, there's a little Bird.
Bird/Glen:	Tweet, tweet. Tweet, tweet.
Mother:	Where's Little Red?
Bird:	Caw, caw!
Mother:	Is something wrong?
Bird:	Caw, caw!
Mother:	All right, I'll follow the little Bird. Is there something wrong?
Bird:	[*Agitated*] Tweet, tweet!
Mother:	Follow you?
Bird:	Tweet, tweet!
Mother:	All right.
Narrator:	So Mother followed the Bird through the woods, past the trees and over the hills and the Bird led her…
Bird:	Caw, caw. Squeal, squeal.
Narrator:	to Grandmother's house.

When Mother (therapist) entered Grandmother's house she discovered both Little Red and Grandmother doing well. Then Glen became the Wolf and proceeded to scare and attack Mother. He then said, 'Ha, ha, you fell for it! It was a joke, to scare you.' The Bird (Glen) returned and explained to Mother all that had happened in 'bird language,' a combination of high-pitched squeals and English. Then the Wolf returned again to scare Mother, as a 'joke.' Then the Bird began frenzied squealing, indicating the Wolf's mother was coming. The Bird killed the Wolf's mother and left 'blood on the knife.' Mother thanked the Bird with a bowl of worms.

Once again, Glen was playing opposing forces, counter-roles. He was the frenzied little Bird and the Wolf's mother, who was angrier than the original Wolf: the small and helpless role and the all-powerful and destructive role, simultaneously. The small and weak Bird overcame great obstacles in defeating the recurring role of the Wolf or Wolf's mother. Glen chose to repeatedly scare Little Red's Mother, later saying it was all a joke. When Glen's own Mother was asked during an interview whether she felt Glen's medical condition caused stress, she replied, 'I think, yeah, especially as a baby, from zero to four years. For the family, it was very scary' (Mrs D, personal communication, September 26 1997). During this particular dramatization, Glen chose to repeatedly scare 'Mother' in an unpredictable manner, only to justify his actions by reneging on his original intentions.

Glen's favorite projective technique was make-up. During *The Three Little Pigs*, the story he selected most often, he used brown face make-up as the 'mud.' He also added green make-up to represent grass stains where the Pigs fell in the grass. Although he applied make-up as the Pig characters, he would also play the Wolf. Glen always took both sides of a struggle. His favorite part was the 'whole story.' His favorite role was the 'oldest Pig.' When asked by the therapist, Glen stated he wanted to be the 'three boys.'

So, during the eighth session, with the story progressing, Glen played all roles, save that of Mother.

Narrator / Therapist:	So, the mean Wolf walked over to the house of straw and said:
Wolf / Glen:	Ahhh! Knock, knock. Open up.
Pig / Glen:	Not by the hair of my chinny chin chin.
Wolf:	Or I'll huff and I'll blow your house down.
Pig:	Not by the hair of my chinny chin chin.
Wolf:	All right.
Narrator / Glen:	And he huffed [*takes deep, difficult breath and blows*] and he blew the house down. Then he gobbled 'em all up. Then he went to the next house.
Wolf:	Knock, knock.
Pig:	Who is it?
Wolf:	Open up!
Pig:	Not by the hair of my chinny chin chin.
Wolf:	Then I'll huff and I'll blow your house down.

Pig:	Not by the hair of my chinny chin chin.
Wolf:	All right.
Narrator:	[*Whispers*] So he huffed [*takes a breath*] and he puffed [*builds*] and blew the house down.
Wolf:	Now open up.
Pig:	Not by the hair of my chinny chin chin.

The story repeats. Each time the Wolf's huffing and puffing becomes labored. He tries repeatedly to blow down the brick house and cannot.

Wolf:	What is up with this house, yo?

Glen's repetition of the Wolf's breathing is not only labored but appears to be frustrating, as well. According to Glen's social worker:

Prednisone shrinks inflammation and tissue, you know? So it's everything about him, especially his lungs, that...well, he had to have chest PT (physical therapy), where they pound on his chest, because the stuff was all inside of his lungs. He gets really bad. He's got a very serious illness. (JM, personal communication, September 18 1997)

The Wolf's breathing is his means for survival. Not just natural breathing, but a breath so strong it can blow down houses. When the Wolf's breath fails him, he winds up drowning in a bubbling pot. As was previously noted, an asthmatic may have a fear of dying by suffocation (O'Dougherty and Brown 1990). In the case of *The Three Little Pigs*, the Wolf does die by drowning or suffocating in the bubbling pot. As the Wolf lands in the pot, Glen lets out a blood-curdling scream.

The Children's Manifest Anxiety Scale – Revised (CMAS-R) was administered to Glen as both a pre- and post-test. Glen's pre-test score was 19, well above the mean of 13.84, indicating a high anxiety/stress level at the beginning of the treatment. Glen's post-test score was 20. The CMAS-R did not suggest a reduction in Glen's stress level, although because of his young age of seven, it is not considered a reliable measure. Unbeknown to the therapist, the last few dramatherapy sessions had been scheduled by his teacher during Glen's recess period, since school had begun again. This may have had an adverse effect on Glen's stress level.

The CMAS-R results were surprising as Glen had the highest scores of any of the experimental subjects, both for the pre- and post-test. Staff members had referred to Glen as being well adjusted, yet his scores seemed to indicate otherwise. Although Glen appeared to be happy, he may have been experiencing stress due to his illness.

Overall, the dramatherapy sessions appeared to be very productive for Glen. He was always eager and well motivated. Glen actively participated by becoming several roles, including counter-roles, and often even the narrator. Glen always played counter-roles, such as Jack and the Giant, or the three little Pigs and the Wolf. Glen attempted to achieve a balance by exploring such opposing forces. Glen's need to become opposing forces in each story was reflective of his living in the ambivalence.

The issues Glen presented through the role-playing suggested a fear of death, and separation anxiety. Glen had experienced several recent deaths in his family, as well as being hospitalized himself due to the severity of his condition. In addition to focusing on many death-related scenes within the fairy tales themselves, Glen also created several aged characters. A 7-year-old boy, choosing to put wrinkles and age spots on his otherwise swollen face, through the use of the stage make-up, is rare – especially old-age characters that otherwise were never specified as such. Glen needed to become old through the role-playing. According to Glen's mother: 'He really liked it [dramatherapy]. He thought it was really cool. I think it was good. It opened him up creatively. He loved it. He would come home and act out the stories he did' (Mrs D, personal communication, September 20 1997).

Glen's enjoyment of this creative modality appeared to fuel his motivation. According to Glen's mother, he also became more motivated around the house, actually volunteering to do chores, since his dramatherapy treatment. Based on the observational stress measure and the feedback from staff, Glen was initially presented as being happy. However, as the CMAS-R suggested, Glen did have a relatively high level of stress/anxiety. It appeared as though his stress may have been hidden behind a happy facade. The combination of Glen's severe asthma and weight gains almost doubling his young poundage can produce stress. When his weight went up, he was conscious of it.

Overall, it appears as though the dramatherapy sessions were very productive for Glen and that his stress level may have been reduced. Glen's weight was reduced back to his original 60 pounds, having lost almost 40 pounds. He was weaned off the prednisone over the course of the summer, while engaging in the dramatherapy treatment. Glen now weighed 60 pounds, rather than 100 pounds. Glen's having repeatedly played the role of the hero/Pig from *The Three Little Pigs* may have been his way of adding strength of character and dignity to an otherwise stereotypically plump glutton.

Six-Month Follow-Up

Glen greatly improved over the last six months. Although this was considered to be a 'bad year for asthma,' he avoided any unscheduled hospitalizations. According to his nurse, Glen's health had improved for the first time since he was admitted to this partial hospitalization program (DS, personal communication, March 23 1998).

Glen doesn't indicate any overt symptoms of stress, according to his primary nurse, but rather is considered to be 'even keel...a typical third grader' (ML, personal communication, March 23 1998). Glen's physicians and treatment team are discussing a possible discharge, yet the program doesn't advocate releasing a patient in the middle of a school semester. Not only has Glen's condition greatly improved and his stress is seemingly managed, but Glen was elected as mayor of the partial hospitalization program. The role of mayor is one for which Glen has always strived.

Transcript of selected session
Glen: Selected Session #6 (9/4/97)

Therapist:	We're here today for Drama with Miss Carol, that's myself, and Glen. Glen, would you like to say hello to everyone?
Glen:	Hello.

Therapist:	We're planning to act out a story for you today. As always we'll have the selection of five stories. Let's continue.
Therapist:	For today, Glen, you can select from five stories and I'll be planning to meet you as we did during the summer, Tuesdays and Thursdays, beginning today. The selection of the stories are: *Hansel and Gretel, Jack and the Beanstalk, Little Red Riding Hood, The Gingerbread Man* or *The Three Little Pigs.*
Glen:	What story is it that I didn't do yet?
Therapist:	Do you want me to check my list? I have the master list.
Glen:	Let's see what stories I already did.
Therapist:	You haven't done – you didn't do *Hansel and Gretel.*
Glen:	*Hansel and Gretel?* I'll do that one.
Therapist:	OK?
Glen:	Uh huh.
Therapist:	I'll begin by telling you the story and then we'll continue from there. This is the story called *Hansel and Gretel.* A long time ago and very far away, there lived a little boy and a little girl named Hansel and Gretel [*acts out story for Glen*].
Therapist:	And then Hansel and Gretel…
Glen:	…lived happily ever after.
Narrator:	And that's the story of Hansel and Gretel.
Therapist:	Now then – if you could be anyone in the story of Hansel and Gretel, who would you choose to be?
Glen:	Ummm – ummmm – ummmm – ummmm – ummmm. Let me see. The little boy and the guy and you can be the little girl and the girl. OK?
Therapist:	OK. And what part of the story would you like to do? The whole story? Or part of the story?
Glen:	The whole story.
Therapist:	Oh, we have plenty of time. So you're going to be the… OK I've got it.

Glen:	Can we use the walkie-talkie thing?
Therapist:	Yes, we can. If you see if it's handy. You want to hook it right up to here, you mean?
Glen:	Yeah.
Therapist:	OK, here you go. Ready?
Glen:	I will be the guy and the little boy.
Therapist:	I will be the Stepmother and the girl named Gretel.
Glen:	And let's start the thing. Wasn't he a sailor. The guy...I thought he wore a hat in the book.
Therapist:	Yes, that's good. That's very good.
Glen:	And the little boy...
Therapist:	Did you want to put some on today?
Glen:	I'll use this... [*Applies make-up*]. I'll use this brown.
Therapist:	Like you said, from being so poor and playing in the woods. Good. Is this everything? Oh, you look so good. Do you want to look in the mirror?
Glen:	Uh huh. OK. Let's start. *We'll do Hansel and Gretel.*
Therapist:	A long, long time ago and very far away there lived a little boy and girl named Hansel and Gretel. One night while they lay sleeping their Stepmother and Father were having this conversation.
Stepmother / Therapist:	Tomorrow we're taking the children to the woods, we're leaving them there – that's final.
Father / Glen:	But, but...
Stepmother:	Don't give me any but, but. We have no money. We have no food. We've got some bread. So there's really no choice in the matter, is there?
Father:	No. All right.
Stepmother:	All right then. And I don't want to hear another word. We're taking the children and that's final.
Father:	All right.
Narrator / Therapist:	So the next morning Hansel and Gretel went for a walk out in the woods with their Stepmother and Father.

Stepmother:	Go over there and get some sticks. Go on – get some sticks and berries. Make use of yourselves – you simples.
Gretel/Therapist:	I'm worried, Hansel. I'm afraid of what they might do.
Hansel/Glen:	Don't worry. I left bread tracks. I left bread – I left tracks.
Gretel:	Oh you did? You left a track of the bread?
Hansel:	Uh huh.
Narrator/Therapist:	And Stepmother and Father were gone.
Gretel	Oh! They're gone, Hansel, what should we do?
Hansel:	Don't worry. I left tracks.
Gretel:	Oh that was so smart. Hey! Where's the bread? The bird is there!
Bird/Glen:	Caw caw.
Hansel and Gretel:	Shoo, shoo, shoo.
Gretel:	Oh no. What are we going to do now, Hansel?
Hansel:	Hey, look at that house!
Hansel and Gretel:	Let's go!
Narrator/Therapist:	So Hansel and Gretel ran over as fast they could to the gingerbread house [*running footsteps*] and they took a bite.
Gretel:	Ummmmmm…try this! Look, lemon drops. Ummmmmm…sugar gummies.
Hansel:	Oooooh…candy canes.
Narrator/Witch/Therapist/Glen:	So what they didn't know – from inside the house they heard, 'Nibble, nibble, like a mouse. Who's that nibbling on my house?'
Therapist:	And Hansel and Gretel continued to eat.
Hansel and Gretel:	Ummmm…oh my gosh, this is so good! Try this cake! Ummmm…icing, licorice sticks.
Narrator/Therapist:	And then all of a sudden out came an old woman who said…
Witch/Therapist and Glen:	Nibble, nibble, like a mouse. Who's that nibbling at my house. Who is it?

Hansel/Glen: We're sorry. We would repay you if we could.

Witch/Therapist: Ohhhh...dearie, dear. Come right in, my little skinny thing. Sit right here and I will give you a sandwich. Would you like a sandwich — you and your sister? There's a nice sandwich. And some drink? Have two.

Hansel/Glen: [*Chewing and eating.*]

Narrator/Therapist: So Hansel and Gretel ate their sandwiches and drank their drink and were very, very happy.

Witch/Therapist: And then the old woman said, 'Well, my little dear, let's see, you're so thin, how can we plump you up?'

Hansel/Glen: [*Still chewing and saying*] Hi.

Witch/Therapist: I'll say. Right this way. I have something to show you. Come here, my dearie.

Narrator/Therapist: So the old woman opened up the cage and [*loudly says*] pushed Hansel in.

Hansel/Glen: [*Screams and laughs.*]

Narrator/Therapist: [*Laughing says*] and locked it [*claps*].

Witch/Therapist: Now, my dear, show me your arm. Oh! It's skinny. It's skinny like a bone! Just like a stick, I say! Now you! Gretel! Get over here and fix the oven!

Narrator/Therapist: So Gretel walked over, opened the oven and said,

Gretel/Therapist: 'Don't worry Hansel, I'll help us.' She said to the Witch, 'Come here, show me how to use this oven, I'm not sure.'

Witch/Therapist: Oh, you good for nothing.

Narrator/Therapist: So the Witch leaned into the oven and Hansel pushed the door shut, ran over and unlocked the key and Hansel came out and all the cookie children turned into children.

Children/Therapist and Glen: Hurray for Hansel! Hurray for Gretel! You saved our day.

Gretel/Therapist: Quick, Hansel, let's go get the money!

Narrator/Therapist: And they ran up [*running footsteps*] and they got gold and jewels from the Witch and they ran home to tell Mother.

Stepmother/Therapist: What are you children doing here?

Hansel/Glen: Gold, silver, we'll be rich!

Stepmother/Therapist: Where did you get this? Did you steal?

Hansel/Glen: No. Just say we borrowed it.

Stepmother/Therapist: Well, now we'll never be poor again.

Narrator/Therapist: And the Stepmother and the Father and Hansel and Gretel...

Narrator and Glen: Lived happily ever after and they were very rich.

Therapist: Good – very good. Now tell me – did you like that story?

Glen: Yeah.

Therapist: What was your favorite part?

Glen: It was the little boy one.

Therapist: Oh, the part of the little boy, Hansel?

Glen: Uh huh.

Therapist: What did you like about Hansel? OK, look at me [*to remove make-up*].

Glen: When he was putting the breadcrumbs down.

Therapist: Oh, the breadcrumbs?

Glen: Uh huh.

Therapist: And leaving the tracks?

Glen: Uh huh.

Therapist: And that was your favorite part.

Glen: Uh huh.

Therapist: Why did you like that part best?

Glen: Because he was smart enough to do that.

Therapist: He was very smart enough to do that.
                      But then what happened?

Glen: A Bird came and ate them.

Therapist: A Bird came and ate all the breadcrumbs. And how'd that make him feel?

Glen: Sad.

Therapist: Yes, very sad. Because there they were in the middle of the woods, what would they do next?

Therapist: Oh, that came off nicely, because it's the new kind. Let me have one tissue for that [*removing make-up*].
You did such a nice job on the story. You almost know all the words and everything. Did you notice?

Glen: Can we do it again?

CHAPTER 5

Afterthoughts

Chronically ill children, as was revealed during this process, often experience loss and pain. Their daily struggle to survive is exacerbated by an imposing array of restrictions. Everyday life becomes a battleground devoid of the simplest childhood pleasures. Even the routine must not be taken for granted. The children of this study must spend their school hours in a special hospital school program, while experiencing frequent in-patient hospital stays. While their illnesses may be visible, their emotional imbalances are often not.

These children have lost any chance of a normal childhood, and have sometimes come close to losing their lives. They often experience physical pain, whether it be an Accu-Check needle prick or simply trying to draw a breath. But it is their emotional pain that is often ignored. These ofttimes minimally verbal children need a way to communicate or express these feelings of loss and pain.

The participating chronically ill children were all experiencing inner turmoil relating to their medical conditions. In most cases, their feelings of angst or frustration were left unresolved. The younger children may not have even known the words to express what they were feeling. It is imperative to treat the patients' minds in addition to their physical being. Although the clinical staff of the partial hospital program offered some group and individual therapy, it was based on traditional verbal methods.

Many children's illnesses are aggravated by stress, particularly severe asthma and diabetes. 'Intense, early family stress is now one of five basic risk factors for the development of asthma that have been identified' (Mrazek 1993, p.198). 'Countless diabetic patients and their doctors had noticed that blood-sugar levels rose during stressful times of life, and some researchers had shown that experimental stress could raise blood sugar in diabetic patients' (Surwit 1993, p.131). Stress can be an integral factor in triggering these illnesses, but the illness itself can bring on stress. This study was designed to determine whether a child's stress level could be reduced by his or her involvement in the drama-therapy treatment program. Analyzing the cumulative results of the CMAS-R, the observational stress measure, the interviews, and the case analyses themselves, the dramatherapy sessions appeared to have reduced the patient's level of stress/anxiety. Three of the five study participants had a marked improvement in their health, as was determined by the six-month follow-up interviewing process. Cases 2, 4 and 5 all indicated an improvement in health. Cases 1 and 3 actually had an improvement in their medical conditions immediately following the dramatherapy treatment, but not as of the six-month follow-up. Case 1, however, did show great improvement in health after one year.

The individual dramatherapy sessions provided the children with a non-threatening and inviting manner for self-expression and exploration. The root of the sessions was the use of classic fairy tales. Story making, a powerful means of often symbolic communication, is a natural expression of play for children. 'People who know and love stories will tell anyone: tales are potent stuff – not just the material dreams are made of, but the very substance of humanness' (Gersie 1997, p.13). The children were able to express themselves through the five carefully selected stories. The five stories that had been pre-selected by the therapist based on their issue applicability were very evenly chosen and explored within the therapy sessions (see Appendix B).

The five fairy tales dealt with separation anxiety, loss of control, and a fear of bodily harm or death – the issues previously determined to be the central concern for chronically ill children. Through an analysis of the case studies, including pattern matching and explanation building, all three of these issues were explored by each subject, although the younger children demonstrated a more profound concern for separation anxiety, at least early on in the work. All issues were explored in that each child enacted each of the five stories at least once (see Appendix B). The most prevalent issue within the dramatizations, however, was bodily harm or death. Each of the children has literally faced death, and death was the most central issue within their dramatizations. The threat of death was the most recurring theme.

The role method (Landy 1993) was applied to the cases in an attempt to further assess the functioning of the patient. The role method is a way to decipher the patient's ability to select roles, enact them and then gain personal insight as to their inherent meaning. The seven steps of the role method provided a method for analyzing the dramatherapy treatment. Simply invoking and naming a role is a revealing process. The qualities inherent in the roles can also prove meaningful as they reflect qualities of a patient's life, often strengthening the patient's emotional condition. A child may take on a strong or physically active role because he or she is weak with illness.

The qualities of the roles enacted offer insight into the child's own needs and stymied motivations. Although the patients expressed extensive and detailed qualities, any direct verbal interpretations by the therapist were kept to a minimum. Interpretations or reflections were made within the story or in referring to the story, unless the child was comfortable in reflecting on his or her own. Often with fragile and minimally verbal children, such as this chronically ill population, direct interpretations tend to violate the necessary distance of this modality. With the young age and chronic condition of the patients, the therapist was able to analyze and interpret each case based on the role method.

The exploration of the counter-roles proved insightful. This is Landy's more recent criterion for assessment (R. Landy, personal communication, March 15 1998). In some cases (Case 1 and Case 4) the roles were clearly focused, such as the role of the Bird and the Wolf. However, in the other three cases, each patient actually explored counter-roles at the same time, acting out the roles of the protagonist and the antagonist within a single session. The explorations of counter-roles can indicate a search for balance, which is necessary for wellness. If a child didn't explore a counter-role, it may have been because his or her need to connect with one preferred role was paramount. This may have been a reflection of a personal imbalance. The children who repetitively focused on a single role did so for a compelling reason (see Appendix B).

The qualities and counter-qualities of each role proved valuable in suggesting meaning, as did the function and aesthetic distance of the roles. The wide repertoire of roles that patients invoked were examined according to the quality, function and style as depicted in the taxonomy of roles described by Landy. Patterns were explored (see Appendix B) and discoveries made. The roles only came to life when a child made a selection, becoming specifically designed for each individual child, although as the story originally unfolded they were generic. But as the child and the role became one, the role took on the child's fears and processed it. The role had the strength to carry the self and in this sense took the player on a journey of discovery.

The connection between fiction and everyday life is the essence of dramatherapy. Fragile children are able to express themselves through storymaking, and in what seems to them to be playing they can strive for understanding. Although this understanding is often unspoken or even unconscious, it is still communicated through a combination of symbols and emotions, with positive results. Dramatic role-playing is a natural and non-threatening form of expression for children. Fairy tales are familiar yet powerful stories for therapy. These elements, when presented to children who can't or won't speak about their emotional conflicts, can prove to be very successful for treatment. It is the power of the children's own fiction that reflects lives and provides them with an opportunity to examine and improve their situation. A child can soar like a bird to experience a freedom she'll never know or a child can become death itself in order to face her darkest fears. Through drama, these children can pretend so they may improve their reality through this escape into fiction. Any long-term effects may relate to the longevity of the treatment process.

One of the most powerful discoveries the therapist made involved how the children's physical limitations were faced or played out through the dramatizations. In Case 2, the young girl with diabetes could not stop eating the gingerbread house. In Case 3, the boy with severe asthma could not huff and puff strongly enough to blow down the brick house. Case 1 revealed that the young girl with the oxygen tank attached to her as a means of life support was able to fly through the role of the Bird. Through the dramatherapy, the children were able to overcome their physical burdens, if only for a moment and if only through the use of their imaginations.

This dramatherapy program had several integral components that led to its success. The partial day program being that of an actual school housed in a hospital provided a model atmosphere. If the work had been conducted with a chronic in-patient population of a pediatric unit, the children may have been at times too sick to participate. A pediatric unit can also be conducive to many interruptions by assigned medical staff and has the potential for the imminent discharge of its patients. Out-patient therapy would have had possible scheduling or commitment problems. The hospital/school setting was an ideal environment to conduct the dramatherapy sessions.

Conducting individual rather than group dramatherapy sessions provided for a solid foundation. Individual therapy allows for the client or patient to indulge completely in his or her unresolved conflicts. It affords the client all of the attention and makes them feel special (JM, personal communication, September 18 1997). Some of these chronically ill children were fragile, and in some cases, because of their passivity or self-consciousness in expressing themselves, would not feel comfortable within a group dynamic. The case study method allowed the researcher to make a detailed analysis of each individual.

The CMAS-R, the stress measure and the interviews all provided valuable and much-needed information. Insight shared by various staff members and by the parents of the children provided explanatory background detail. However, the most significant source of information remained the dramatherapy sessions themselves. The spontaneous and improvisational-based dramatizations illuminated the child's conscious or unconscious fears and desires. The most difficult part of this work was to capture the power of the artistry that was created within any given moment of self-expression and convey it through mere words.

An audiotape recorder proved invaluable in documenting all verbal communications during the sessions. Videotaping was rejected in order that the patient would feel less threatened. Another consideration was whether to photograph the children as they wore their make-up. The make-up designs were so original and painstakingly symbolic, it would have been helpful to the reader if anonymous photographs had been included in the text. The decision not to photograph the children was based on their need for privacy and anonymity. Any photographs could have been reproduced graphically, in order to maintain the child's privacy. However, photographing children during a therapy session may have been intrusive and detrimental to the patient's feelings of privacy.

Beyond these aforementioned variables, it is vital for the drama-therapist to have the ability to step into the child's world of imagination. The therapist must suspend disbelief and enter into the realm of dramatic play. Without this capability the work is futile. Communicating with a child through his or her own language of play is paramount in establishing a therapeutic bond and a healing connection. A dramatherapist needs to be skilled in the art of acting and as a clinician. It is the merging of both of these roles that is required, although the healing occurs within the artistry itself.

Further research or practice in this area, beyond the scope of this present work, should be considered. Variables to explore include increasing the number of patients or extending the treatment time. The length of treatment time could be longer; however, shorter psychotherapeutic treatment is currently being promoted in the mental health community. Future studies or practice could encourage a child's own original story to be enacted, instead of, or in addition to, provided fairy tales. The children of this study had available a variety of puppets, masks, make-up and costume accessories, which enhanced role-playing. Some practitioners may want to isolate the use of certain techniques.

It appears as though dramatherapy may reduce stress in children and therefore promote mind and body healing. This study has suggested a relationship between dramatherapy treatment and stress reduction. Stress is an integral factor in chronic illness. Future studies may link dramatherapy to an improvement in medical conditions, in part because of the stress reduction that can result. This work suggested that dramatherapy can improve mental health when applied to the treatment of hospitalized children.

According to psychiatrist Dr Michael Gunter: 'It is not surprising that most of our childhood patients in isolation treatment on the BMT (bone marrow transplantation) ward have vivid fantasies of flight ...

those children who no longer had fantasies of flight or who merely exhibited fantasies of unsuccessful escape (through art therapy), were the ones who demonstrated extreme stress reactions' (2000). Dr Gunter goes on to explain how the psychic equilibrium is threatened by illness, yet can be overcome through the creative process. The flight motif, which was a recurring pattern in this study as well, is clearly significant. This symbolism should be considered in future research.

Future research in dramatherapy with pediatric populations would be beneficial to the field. Dramatherapy research with any population of children is lacking in the literature. Chronically ill children have an unmet need to explore unresolved emotional issues in a non-threatening manner. It is necessary for a chronically ill child to be healed physically, emotionally, and spiritually. Dramatherapy treatment may actually have a positive effect on the child's medical health. Further research could examine the relationship between dramatherapy intervention and its effect on the chronic illness itself. The new field of Arts Medicine is in need of research to determine the effectiveness of such modalities as dramatherapy. Dramatherapy with pediatric populations is a very new, yet natural, form of healing.

Drama became a universal form of communication for the children that we came to know through this book. The children's chronic illnesses and frailties were not obstacles to their dramatic expression. Their minimal verbalizations or inaudible speech problems were overcome through this newfound ability to communicate within the therapy sessions. The children did not necessarily know they were participating in therapy, or that they were expressing their innermost fears. The patients were not aware that the drama experience might have been a factor in their stress reduction. But the children felt the healing power of the drama on an unconscious level. This was indicated by increased motivation and passion for each subsequent session.

Children of the school/hospital who were not a part of the study asked to have drama too. One young boy, of about the age of eight, who was suffering from a rare and chronic skin disorder that covered most of his frail body, reached up from his wheelchair and grabbed my hand as I walked by. 'Oh, please,' he begged as he held on to my hand, 'can I please come to drama, too?' His skin was so debilitated that I initially thought he was suffering from second or third degree burns. This boy's yearning for drama, his innate need for self-exploration of inner turmoil, clearly is reflective of an unmet need.

Chronically ill children face a grave reality that exists for them daily. Through the safety of a fairy tale, these children can tackle insurmountable and life-threatening dangers with positive results. By exploring an extensive array of conflicting emotions, these children can willingly face tragedy. The Giant doesn't devour them, the Wolf doesn't gobble them up, and the Witch doesn't roast them. They fought the battle against the odds, and they won. It is because of the children's ability to transport themselves to a universal yet timeless place within the tale that they can dare to keep their spirits alive.

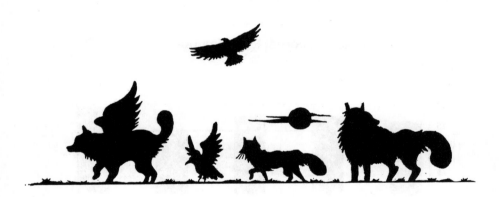

Figure 5.1 They fought the battle against the odds, and they won (illustration by Laurence Muleh 2001)

Appendix A

Results: The Children's Manifest Anxiety Scale – Revised

The Children's Manifest Anxiety Scale – Revised (CMAS-R) was the standardized psychological instrument utilized for this study. Twenty-eight anxiety and nine lie items were administered to ten subjects, five members of the experimental group and five members of a control group. The subjects of the control group were each administered two trials of the CMAS-R, pre-test and post-test, and received no dramatherapy intervention.

Results, including mean scores and standard deviation scores, were compared within and between the experimental and control groups. In addition, mean and standard deviation scores for the subjects in this study were compared with those of the original studies ($N = 167$) by the authors (Reynolds and Richmond 1978).

The pre-test results of the experimental group yielded a group mean of 16.6 for the 28 anxiety items with a standard deviation of 1.8. The mean lie scale score (see p.237) was 4.8, with a standard deviation of 2.3. Post-test results following the ten sessions of dramatherapy indicated a significant decrease on the anxiety scale, with a mean score of 12.8 and a standard deviation of 6.1. Thus, the desired effect of reducing anxiety/stress was achieved for the experimental group (Figure A.1).

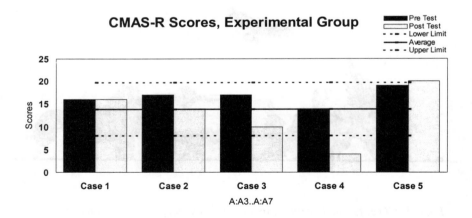

In contrast, mean pre-test score of the control group was 14.2 with a standard deviation of 5.2. Post-test scores for this group were 15.2 with a standard deviation 4.8; no significant change. The control group pre-tested at 3.0 lie scale and 5.8 on the post-test. Clearly, the experimental group reduced anxiety scores, while the control group remained stable or even increased their stress levels (Figure A.2).

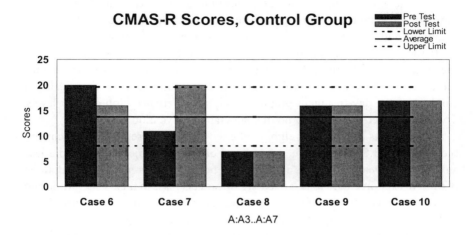

The authors found from their previous studies, based on a larger sample group (N = 167), the mean for the 28 anxiety items was 13.84 with a standard deviation of 5.79. The mean lie scale score that the authors found for large groups was 3.56 with a standard deviation of 2.37 (Reynolds and Richmond 1978). Findings from this study, with its small number of subjects, are consistent with these published results.

This suggests that the therapeutic effect of the intervention reduces stress, but also points up the broad diversity of possible reactions to the intervention. Four of the five subjects in the experiment decreased their anxiety score or maintained it at the initial level. One subject slightly increased his anxiety scale score, but by less than one standard deviation from the pre-test score. With a small sample, only extreme scores can influence the mean as well as the standard deviation of the sample.

For the purposes of this study, the means and standard deviations of the CMAS-R are used to set the parameters of high versus low scores. These scores are on both the anxiety items and the lie items of the scale. The sample size of the current study may limit reliability of statistical references from the subjects in this case study alone. Any score that is more than one standard deviation above the mean, based on the author's calculations, is considered a high score (19.63). Scores that are more than one standard deviation below the mean are considered to be low scores (8.05) on the anxiety items of the CMAS-R. For lie score items, scores of more than one standard deviation above the mean (5.93) are considered high, while scores of more than one standard deviation below the mean (1.19) are considered to be low scores. This indicates the absence of 'faking' an impression in either direction.

Of the five children in the experimental group, all had initial pre-test scores above those in the author's group as is related to the anxiety items. The post-test scores of the experimental group indicate that two of the five subjects had scores below the author's group mean and one was within a single point.

In the pre-test for the control group, three of the five subjects had scores above the mean. Four of the five subjects in this group posted scores above the mean for the post-test. This may be explained because the subjects were chronically ill children of the day treatment program likely to experience high anxiety levels. These five subjects were given no dramatherapy intervention.

These results indicate that eight of the ten subjects presented a high anxiety score (above 13.84) during the pre-test and only three subjects presented a low anxiety score (below 13.84) as a result of the post-test. As previously stated, three of the five experimental subjects had a significant decrease in their score, while one subject remained the same. Only one subject of the five within the control group had a decrease in anxiety and this score was still above average.

The decrease in anxiety represented by the experimental group's cumulative post-test scores indicates a reduction of 19 points following the dramatherapy treatment. The control group increased by five points. The cumulative average of the experimental group's post-test scores was below the author's average (12.80<13.84), a significant reduction from the experimental group's cumulative pre-test average of 16.60. In the published literature, this average is considered high. The control group's cumulative pre-test scores were above average at 14.20 and increased to 15.20 in the post-test. Both the individual scores and the cumulative scores of the experimental group indicate that the dramatherapy intervention was successful in reducing the stress/anxiety of the subjects. This conclusion is further validated by the control group's demonstrating above-average anxiety that increased slightly as a result of having no dramatherapy intervention.

The average of the lie score for the pre-test of the experimental group was 4.8. The post-test lie score average was 4.6. This constancy hovered just above the average of the author's mean lie score of 3.56, further validating the results. The control group's lie score did nearly double from 3.0 to 5.8, which is considered high. This increase could be a result of familiarity with the anxiety items, which enabled the subjects to make more of an attempt to 'fake good' and 'fake bad.' In summary, the subjects of the experimental group showed a decrease in their anxiety and the control group did not.

According to clinical psychologist Dr Cynthia Wiles: 'Descriptive statistics are the method of choice for a qualitative case study' (personal communication, March 25 1998). A t-test or other instrumental measures designed to ensure statistical validity were not deemed necessary for this case study with its small samples (N =

10). Had the sample size been larger (N = 25 <) the student's t-test would have been necessary to assess the results of the scale utilized.

Cumulative analysis of CMAS-R results indicate that the experimental group had a reduction in stress as a result of the dramatherapy intervention. The control group indicated little or no change in stress. According to the staff psychologist, the fact that such a small sample size led to these positive results is highly significant and impressive (TK, personal communications, September 23 1998). The dramatherapy intervention was successful in reducing stress. The following are brief summaries of the three individual case results.

Caitlin

The stress measure (Antoni 1993) was utilized with each patient. The therapist used this observational checklist after the second session, and again after the tenth session. Cognitive, emotional, behavioral, and physiological symptoms were rated on a 1–5 index. For Caitlin, all stress indicators such as poor concentration, restlessness, and avoidance of tasks, were initially marked at 4–5, the highest rating. By the last session, all symptoms had been reduced to the 1–2 range, suggesting Caitlin's stress was reduced. Caitlin's CMAS-R score of 16 remained the same for both tests, indicating no change in stress levels. For the CMAS-R, 13.84 is the mean score, therefore 16 is considered to be above average. This indicated that Caitlin's stress level is somewhat above average. Caitlin's lie score was 7 (pre) and 8 (post), whereas 3.56 is the mean.

A lie scale is a validity scale that indicates how honestly the subjects are responding to the actual items being tested. It is a series of statements that aren't part of the actual test, yet interjected within, so as to appear as such. Any lie score above 5.93 is considered high. Caitlin's score of 8 is very high. 'With younger children a high [lie] score may be interpreted as a measure of social desirability, which could account for the high scores of the grade 1 pupils.' (Reynolds and Richmond 1978). They say that standardized tests with very young children with language disorders or learning disabilities may or may not prove satisfactory:

> A frequent complaint of teachers administering the scale is that...some words are too difficult for primary grade children, slow learners, and the mentally retarded. These groups of children are often the ones whose level of anxiety we seek most to understand. (Reynolds and Richmond 1978, p.272)

According to the results of Caitlin's CMAS-R scores, her young age and the high results of her lie score, her overall results may be less valid than a similar test given to an older child with a lower lie scale score. This could explain why there was no change in Caitlin's seemingly high stress level according to the CMAS-R. This is why additional qualitative measures were utilized in this study. All the scores from each case were discussed cumulatively and in comparison to the control group at the start of this appendix.

Tasha

The stress measure indicates an improvement in Tasha's stress level. The therapist administered this symptomatic checklist after the second session, and again after the tenth session. As was stated, cognitive, emotional, behavioral, and physiological symptoms, which are observable, were rated on a 1–5 scale. Tasha's results indicate that almost all stress-related symptoms showed a marked reduction. All stress indicators such as deficient memory, inability to relax, and fidgeting were initially scored at 3–4, which is the middle-to-high range, but by the last session had been markedly reduced to the lowest rating of 1. This scale suggests that Tasha's stress was significantly reduced.

Tasha's pre-test score was 17, which is above the average score of 13.84. Tasha's post-test score was 14, which is very near the average, and indicates a reduction in anxiety. According to the CMAS-R, Tasha's stress and anxiety levels were reduced, from an above average level to an average level. Tasha's lie score was 5 for the pre-test and 6 for the post-test, which is considered to be above the average of 3.56, but not high. Her pre- and post-test lie scores are consistent, which further validates the results. Tasha's three-point reduction was discussed cumulatively with all experimental subjects and control group scores.

Brandon

The stress measure was administered to Brandon by the therapist after both the second and tenth session. All symptoms were rated on a 1–5 index. Brandon's results indicated an overall decrease in stress-related symptoms after participating in the dramatherapy sessions. Brandon's behavioral and cognitive symptoms had a slight decrease, but were already rated low (level 1–2) during the first administration. More prominent were the emotional and physiological symptoms, which had a greater decrease due to the initially higher rating. The only symptom to increase was the headache/nausea, stomachache symptom due to Brandon's reported physical illness during the ninth session. Overall, the stress measure suggested that there was a reduction in Brandon's stress level.

The CMAS-R was administered as both a pre- and post-test to Brandon. His pre-test score was 17, which is above average. His post-test score was 10, indicating a great reduction in stress. The mean or average score for the CMAS-R is 13.84. Brandon's lie score remained the same, with a score of just 1 for both the pre- and post-test, which adds further validity to Brandon's results. Brandon's CMAS-R results indicated a reduction in stress with a 7-point decrease from the first session to the last.

Appendix B: Story/Role Selection

Table B.1 Story selection per session

Session	Caitlin	Brandon	Tasha
1	Introduction	Introduction	Introduction
2	The Three Little Pigs	Jack and the Beanstalk	Little Red Riding Hood
3	The Gingerbread Man	The Gingerbread Man	Hansel and Gretel
4	Little Red Riding Hood	Hansel and Gretel	Little Red Riding Hood
5	The Three Little Pigs	The Three Little Pigs	Hansel and Gretel
6	Little Red Riding Hood	Little Red Riding Hood	Hansel and Gretel
7	Hansel and Gretel	Jack and the Beanstalk	The Three Little Pigs
8	Jack and the Beanstalk	Hansel and Gretel	Jack and the Beanstalk
9	Jack and the Beanstalk	The Gingerbread Man	Little Red Riding Hood
10	Jack and the Beanstalk	Hansel and Gretel	The Three Little Pigs

Session	Aaron	Glen
1	Introduction	Introduction
2	The Three Little Pigs	The Three Little Pigs
3	Hansel and Gretel	The Gingerbread Man
4	Jack and the Beanstalk	Jack and the Beanstalk
5	Little Red Riding Hood	Little Red Riding Hood
6	The Gingerbread Man	Hansel and Gretel
7	The Gingerbread Man	Jack and the Beanstalk
8	The Gingerbread Man	The Three Little Pigs
9	The Gingerbread Man	Litttle Red Riding Hood
10	The Gingerbread Man	The Three Little Pigs

Coding:

Little Red Riding Hood	Least amount of death/bodily harm references or occurrences
The Three Little Pigs	
The Gingerbread Man	to
Hansel and Gretel	
Jack and the Beanstalk	Most amount of death/bodily harm references or occurrences

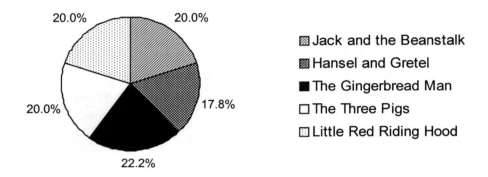

Figure B.1 Subject's story selection (out of 45 stories)

Table B.2 Role selection per session

	Caitlin	Brandon	Tasha
1	Introduction	Introduction	Introduction
2	Mother Pig/Oldest Pig	Jack	Little Red Riding Hood
3	Gingerbread Man	Gingerbread Man	Hansel and Gretel
4	Little Red's Mother/Bird	Hansel and Gretel	Little Red Riding Hood
5	Bird	3 Pigs and Wolf	Hansel and Gretel
6	Bird	Wolf	Gingerbread Man
7	Bird	Jack and Giant	Oldest Pig
8	Bird	Hansel and Gretel	Jack
9	Bird	Gingerbread Man	Wolf/Skeleton
10	Bird	Hansel and Gretel	Oldest Pig/Wolf/Skeleton

Preferred role: Auxiliary (helper)	Preferred role: Protagonist (hero)	Preferred role: Protagonist (hero)

Session	Aaron	Glen
1	Introduction	Introduction
2	Wolf	Wolf/Pigs
3	Witch	Farmer/Wolf
4	Giant	Jack/Giant
5	Wolf	Little Red/Wolf
6	Wolf	Hansel/Father
7	Wolf	Jack/Giant
8	Wolf	Pigs/Wolf
9	Wolf	Little Red/Grandmother
10	Wolf	Pigs/Wolf

<table>
<tr><td>Preferred role:
Antagonist
(beast)</td><td>Preferred role:
Antagonist/protagonist
(beast/hero)</td></tr>
</table>

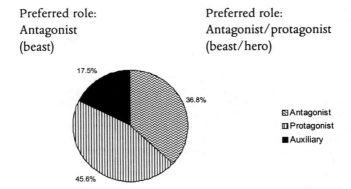

Figure B.2 Subject's role selection

Character coding	
Character:	Type:
Wolf, Witch, Giant, Wolf/Skeleton	Antagonist
Jack, Hansel and Gretel, Little Red, Gingerbread Man, Oldest Pig	Protagonist
3 Pigs and Wolf, Jack and Giant, Oldest Pig/Wolf/Skeleton, Wolf/Pigs	Antagonist/protagonist
Little Red's Mother/Bird, Bird	Auxiliary
Mother Pig/Oldest Pig, Hansel/Father, Little Red/Grandmother	Auxiliary/protagonist
Farmer/Wolf	Auxiliary/antagonist

References

Andrews, T. (1993) *Animal-Speak: The Spiritual and Magical Powers of Creatures Great and Small*. St. Paul, MN: Llewellyn.

Antoni, M. (1993) 'Stress management: Strategies that work.' In D. Goleman and J. Gurin (eds) *Mind and Body Medicine*. New York: Consumers Union.

Axline, V. M. (1947) *Play Therapy*. New York: Houghton Mifflin.

Baker, S. (1993) *Picturing the Beast*. New York: Manchester University Press.

Bartley, M. A. (1997) 'Creativity and medicine: an atelier in medical school.' *International Journal of Arts Medicine 5*, 2, 36–39.

Barton, B. and Booth, D. (1990) *Stories in the Classroom: Storytelling, Reading Aloud, and Role-Playing with Children*. London: Heinemann.

Bettelheim, B. (1975) *The Uses of Enchantment: The Meaning and Importance of Fairy Tales*. New York: Vintage Books.

Bolton, G. (1984) *Drama as Education*. London: Longman.

Bolton, G. (1998) *Acting in Classroom Drama: A Critical Analysis*. London: Trentham Books.

Bornstein, E. M. (1988) 'Therapeutic storytelling.' In R. Zahourek (ed) *Relaxation and Imagery*. Philadelphia, PA: W. B. Saunders.

Briggs, K. (1967) *The Fairies in Tradition and Literature*. London: Routledge.

British Association for Dramatherapists (1979) 'Statement of Goals.' *Drama Therapy 2*, 19.

Brun, B., Pedersen, E. W. and Runberg, M. (1993) *Symbols of the Soul: Therapy and Guidance through Fairy Tales*. London: Jessica Kingsley Publishers.

Campbell, J. (1958) *The Flight of the Wild Gander*. Chicago, IL: Regnery.

Campbell, J. (1972) *Myths to Live By*. New York: Penguin.

Castaneda, A., McCandless, B. and Palermo, D. (1956) 'The Children's Form of the Manifest Anxiety Scale.' *Child Development 27*, 317–326.

Cattanach, A. (1992a) *Play Therapy with Abused Children*. London: Jessica Kingsley Publishers.

Cattanach, A. (1992b) *Drama for People with Special Needs*. New York: Drama Book Publishers.

Cattanach, A. (1997) *Children's Stories in Play Therapy*. London: Jessica Kingsley Publishers.

Chetwynd, T. (1982) *Dictionary of Symbols*. London: Thorsons.

Committee on Child Psychiatry (1982) *The Process of Child Therapy* (no. III, vol. XI). New York: Brunner/Mazel.

Courtney, R. (1980) *The Dramatic Curriculum*. New York: Drama Book Specialists.

Courtney, R. (1989) *Play, Drama and Thought*. New York: Drama Book Specialists.

Eiser, C. (1990) *Chronic Childhood Disease*. Cambridge: Cambridge University Press.

Elliott, C. H., Jay, S. M. and Willis, D. J. (1982) 'Psychological Effects of Physical Illness and its Concomitant.' In J. M. Tuma (ed) *Handbook for the Practice of Pediatric Psychology*. New York: Wiley.

Emunah, R. (1994) *Acting for Real*. New York: Brunner/Mazel.

Fox, J. (1987) *The Essential Moreno*. New York: Springer.

Freud, A. (1966) *The Ego and the Mechanisms of Defense*. Connecticut: International Universities Press.

Gersie, A. (1991) *Storymaking in Bereavement: Dragons Fight in the Meadows*. London: Jessica Kingsley Publishers.

Gersie, A. (1993) *Earth Tales*. London: Jessica Kingsley Publishers.

Gersie, A. (1997) *Reflections on Therapeutic Storymaking*. London: Jessica Kingsley Publishers.

Gersie, A. and King, N. (1990) *Storymaking in Education and Therapy*. London: Jessica Kingsley Publishers.

Golden, D. (1983) 'Play Therapy for Hospitalized Children.' In C. Schaefer and K. O'Connor (eds) *The Handbook of Play Therapy*. New York: Wiley.

Gunter, M. (2000) 'Art Therapy as an Intervention to Stabilize the Defenses of Children Undergoing Bone Marrow Transplantation.' *The Arts in Psychotherapy 27*, 1, 3–14.

Haase, D. (1993) 'Motifs: Making Fairy Tales Our Own.' In G. Blatt (ed) *Once Upon a Folktale*. New York: Teacher's College Press.

Handoo, J. (1990) 'Cultural Attitudes to Birds and Animals in Folklore.' In R. Willis (ed) *Signifying Animals: Human Meaning in the Natural World*. London: Unwin Hyman.

Heathcote, D. and Bolton, G. (1995) *Drama for Learning: Dorothy Heathcote's Mantle of the Expert Approach to Education*. London: Heinemann.

Heuscher, J. E. (1974) *A Psychiatric Study of Myths and Fairy Tales*. Springfield, IL: Charles C. Thomas.

Irwin, E. (1977) 'Play, Fantasy and Symbols: Drama with Emotionally Disturbed Children.' *American Journal of Psychotherapy 31*, 3.

Irwin, E. (1983) 'The Diagnostic and Therapeutic Use of Pretend Play.' In C. Schaefer and K. O'Connor (eds) *The Handbook of Play Therapy*. New York: Wiley.

Jacoby, M., Kast, V. and Riedel, I. (1992) *Witches, Ogres and the Devil's Daughter: Encounters with Evil in Fairy Tales*. Boston, MA: Shambhala.

Jennings, S. (1986) *Creative Drama in Group Work*. London: Winslow Press.

Jennings, S. (ed) (1987) *Drama Therapy: Theory and Practice for Teachers and Clinicians*. London: Croom Helm.

Jennings, S. (1990) *Drama Therapy with Families, Groups and Individuals: Waiting in the Wings*. London: Jessica Kingsley Publishers.

Jennings, S. (1993) *Play Therapy with Children*. Oxford: Blackwell.

Jennings, S. (1998) *Introduction to Drama Therapy: Theatre and Healing*. London: Jessica Kingsley Publishers.

Jones, S. (1995) *The Fairy Tale: The Magic Mirror and Imagination*. New York: Twayne.

Jung, C. G. (ed) (1964) *Man and His Symbols*. New York: Dell.

King, N. (1993) *Storymaking and Drama*. New Hampshire: Heinemann.

Kovacs, M. and Iyengar, S. (1990) 'Psychological Functioning of Children with Insulin Dependent Diabetes Mellitus.' *Journal of Pediatric Psychology 15*, 619–632.

Landy, R. (1982) *Handbook of Educational Drama and Theatre*. Westport, CT: Greenwood Press.

Landy, R. (1986) *Drama Therapy: Concepts, Theories and Practices*, 1st edn. Springfield, IL: Charles C. Thomas.

Landy, R. (1992) 'A Taxonomy of Roles: A Blueprint for the Possibilities of Being.' *The Arts in Psychotherapy 18*, 419–413.

Landy, R. (1993) *Persona and Performance: The Meaning of Role in Drama, Therapy and Everyday Life*. New York: Guilford Press.

Landy, R. (1994) *Drama Therapy: Concepts Theories and Practices*, 2nd edn. Springfield, IL: Charles C. Thomas.

Leete-Hodge, L. (1983) *The Best Traditional Fairy Stories*. London: Dean's International Publishing.

Lubkin, I. M. (1990) *Chronic Illness: Impact and Interventions*. Boston, MA: Jones and Bartlett.

Mallet, C. (1984) *Fairytales and Children*. New York: Schocken.

Mrazek, D. (1993) 'Asthma: Stress, Allergies, and the Genes.' In D. Goleman and J. Gurin (eds) *Mind Body Medicine*. New York: Consumers Union.

Neelands, J. (1984) *Making Sense of Drama*. London: Heinemann.

O'Dougherty, M. and Brown, R. (1990) 'The Stress of Childhood Illness.' In L. E. Arnold (ed) *Childhood Stress*. New York: John Wiley.

Opie, I. and P. (1974) *The Classic Fairy Tales*. Oxford: Oxford University Press.

Pelletier, K. (1993) 'Between Mind and Body: Stress, Emotions, and Health.' In D. Goleman and J. Gurin (eds) *Mind Body Medicine*. New York: Consumers Union.

Piaget, J. (1962) *Play, Dreams and Imitations in Childhood*. New York: Norton.

Prugh, D. G. (1983) *The Psychosocial Aspects of Pediatrics*. Philadelphia, PA: Lea and Febiger.

Reynolds, C. and Richmond, B. (1978) 'What I Think and Feel: A Revised Measure of Children's Manifest Anxiety.' *Journal of Abnormal Child Psychology 6*, 271–280.

Roberts, M. C. (1986) *Pediatric Psychology*. New York: Pergamon.

Rowland, B. (1973) *Animals with Human Faces. A Guide to Animal Symbolism*. Knoxville: University of Tennessee Press.

Sale, R. (1978) *Fairy Tales and After*. Cambridge: Harvard University Press.

Sax, B. (1990) *The Frog King*. New York: Pace University Press.

Schaefer, C. and O'Connor, K. J. (eds) (1983) *Handbook of Play Therapy*. New York: Wiley.

Siegel, L. (1993) 'Psychotherapy with Medically At Risk Children.' In T. Kratochwill and J. Morris (eds) *Handbook of Psychotherapy with Children and Adolescents*. Boston, MA: Allyn and Bacon.

Siegel, L., Smith, K. and Wood, T. (1991) 'Children Medically at Risk.' In T. Kratochwill and R. Morris (eds) *The Practice of Child Therapy*. New York: Pergamon.

Slade, P. (1954) *Child Drama*. London: University of London Press.

Slade, P. (1995) *Child Play*. Bristol, PA: Taylor and Francis.

Stein, R. (1997) *Healthcare for Children: What's Right, What's Wrong, What's Next?* New York: United Hospital Fund.

Surwit, R. (1993) 'Diabetes: Mind over Metabolism.' In D. Goleman and J. Gurin (eds) *Mind Body Medicine*. New York: Consumers Union.

Tatar, M. (1992) *Off with Their Heads: Fairy Tales and the Culture of Childhood*. Princeton, NJ: Princeton University Press.

Thomas, J. (1989) *Inside the Wolf's Belly*. Sheffield: Sheffield Academic Press.

Von Franz, M. (1987) *Interpretation of Fairy Tales*. Texas: Spring Publications.

Von Franz, M. (1993) *The Feminine in Fairy Tales*. Boston, MA: Shambhala.

Von Franz, M. (1995) *Shadow and Evil in Fairy Tales*. Boston, MA: Shambhala.

Wagner, B. J. (1976) *Dorothy Heathcote: Drama as a Learning Medium*. Washington DC: National Education Association.

Warner, M. (1994) *From the Beast to the Blonde*. London: Chatto and Windus.

Way, B. (1967) *Development through Drama*. London: Longman.

Willis, R. (ed) (1990) *Signifying Animals*. London: Unwin Hyman.

Winnicott, D. W. (1971) *Playing and Reality*. London: Tavistock.

Wojtasik, S. and Sanborn, S. (1991) 'The Crisis of Acute Hospitalization.' In N. Webb (ed) *Play Therapy with Children in Crisis*. New York: Guilford Press.

Zipes, J. (ed) (1991) *Spells of Enchantment: The Wondrous Fairy Tales of Western Culture*. New York: Penguin.

Zipes, J. (ed) (1994) *Fairy Tale as Myth: Myth as Fairy Tale*. Kentucky: Kentucky University Press.

Further Reading

Arnheim, R. (1990) 'The Artist as Healer.' *The Arts in Psychotherapy 17*, 1–4.

Arnold, L. E. (ed) (1983) *Childhood Stress*. New York: Wiley.

Atala, K. D. and Carter, B. D. (1992) 'Pediatric Limb Amputation: Aspects of Coping and Psychotherapeutic Interventions.' *Child Psychiatry and Human Development 23*, 2, 117–130.

Azarnoff, P. and Flegal, S. (1975) *A Pediatric Play Program*. Springfield IL: Charles C. Thomas.

Baker, A. and Greene, E. (1987) *Storytelling: Art and Technique*. New York: R. R. Bowker.

Barchers, S. I. (1990) *Wise Women: Folk and Fairy Tales from around the World*. Colorado: Libraries Unlimited.

Bearison, D. J. (1991) *They Never Want to Tell You: Children Talk about Cancer*. Cambridge, MA: Harvard University Press.

Bennett, E. A. (1967) *What Jung Really Said*. New York: Schocken.

Boal, A. (1995) *Rainbow of Desire*. London: Routledge.

Bottigheimer, R. B. (1987) *Grimm's Bad Girls and Bold Boys: The Moral and Social Vision of the Tales*. New Haven, CT: Yale University Press.

Brand, E. B. (1990) 'Children's Coping with Diabetes.' *Journal of Pediatric Psychology 15*, 27–41.

Brannen, J. (1992) *Mixing Methods: Qualitative and Quantitative Research*. Aldershot: Avebury.

Bretherton, I. (ed) (1984) *Symbolic Play*. New York: Academic Press.

Canton, K. (1994) *The Fairy Tale Revisited*. New York: Peter Lang.

Carpenter, P. (1992) 'Perceived Control as a Predictor of Distress in Children Undergoing Invasive Medical Procedures.' *Journal of Pediatric Psychology 17*, 757–773.

Chandler, L. (1985) *Assessing Stress in Children*. New York: Praeger.

Claflin, C. and Barbarin, O. (1991) 'Does Telling Less Protect More? Relationships among Age, Information Disclosure, and what Children with Cancer See and Feel.' *Journal of Pediatric Psychology 16*, 2, 161–191.

Clancier, A. and Kalmanovitch, J. (1984) *Winnicott and Paradox from Birth to Creation*. New York: Tavistock.

Cohen, D. (1987) *The Development of Play*. New York: Routledge.

Cole, T. and Chinoy, H. K. (1970) *Actors on Acting*. New York: Crown.

Courtney, R. (1987) *The Quest: Research and Inquiry in Arts Education*. New York: University Press of America.

Courtney, R. and Schattner, G. (eds) (1981) *Drama in Therapy*, vols 1 and 2. New York: Drama Book Specialists.

Delpo, E. and Frick, S. (1988) 'Directed and Non-directed Play as Therapeutic Modalities.' *Children's Health Care 16*, 261–267.

Dieckmann, H. (1986) *Twice-Told Tales: The Psychological Use of Fairy Tales*. Wilmette IL: Chiron.

Dunne, P. B. (1988) 'Drama Therapy Techniques in One-to-One Treatment with Disturbed Children and Adolescents.' *The Arts in Psychotherapy 15*, 139–149.

Eiser, C. (1992) 'Adjustment to Chronic Disease in Relation to Age and Gender.' *Journal of Pediatric Psychology 17*, 261–275.

Eliaz, E. (1985) *Transference in Drama Therapy*. Michigan: Dissertation Services.

Fink, S. O. (1990) 'Approaches to Emotion in Psychotherapy and Theatre: Implications for Drama Therapy.' *The Arts in Psychotherapy 17*, 5–18.

Firestone, P., McGrath, P. and Feldman, W. (eds) (1983) *Advances in Behavioral Medicine for Children and Adolescents*. London: Lawrence Erlbaum.

Frame, C. and Matson, J. (eds) (1987) *Handbook of Assessment in Childhood Psychopathology*. New York: Plenum Press.

Francis, G. and Ollendick, T. (1987) 'Anxiety Disorders.' In C. Frame and J. Matson (eds) *Handbook of Assessment in Childhood Psychopathology*. New York: Plenum Press.

Franks, B. and Fraenkel, D. (1991) 'Fairy Tales and Dance/Movement Therapy.' *The Arts in Psychotherapy 18*, 311–319.

Freud, S. (1966) *Introductory Lectures on Psychoanalysis.* New York: Norton.

Gapel, S., Oster, G. and Butnik, S. M. (1986) *Understanding Psychological Testing in Children.* New York: Plenum Medical Book Company.

Gardner, R. A. (1993) *Psychotherapy with Children.* London: Jason Aronson.

Gil, E. (1991) *The Healing Power of Play.* New York: Guilford Press.

Goffman, E. (1959) *The Presentation of Self in Everyday Life.* Garden City: Doubleday.

Hagglund, K. (1994) 'Assessing Anger Expression in Children and Adolescents.' *Journal of Pediatric Psychology 22*, 3, 291–304.

Hamel, J. (1993) *Case Study Methods.* London: Sage.

Hartley, R. E. (1952) *Understanding Children's Play.* New York: Columbia University Press.

Haviland, V. (ed) (1973) *Children and Literature: Views and Reviews.* New York: Lothrop, Lee and Shepard.

Herron, R. E. (1971) *Child's Play.* New York: Wiley.

Hillman, J. (1983) *Healing Fiction.* New York: Station Hill.

Hodgson, J. (ed) (1972) *The Uses of Drama.* London: Methuen.

Hodgson, J. and Richards, E. (1966) *Improvisation.* New York: Grove Press.

Irwin, E. (1985) 'Externalizing and Improvising Imagery through Drama Therapy.' *Journal of Mental Imagery 9*, 33–42.

Jennings, S. (1978) *Remedial Drama.* London: A and C. Black.

Jennings, S. and Minde, A. (1993) *Art Therapy and Drama Therapy: Masks of the Soul.* London: Jessica Kingsley Publishers.

Johnson, A. E. (trans.) (1969) *Perrault's Fairy Tales.* New York: Dover.

Johnson, D. R. (1991) 'The Theory and Technique of Transformations in Drama Therapy.' *The Arts in Psychotherapy 18*, 285–300.

Johnson, J. and Johnson, S. (1991) *Advances in Child Health Psychology.* Gainesville, FL: University of Florida Press.

Johnson, M. R. and Mesibov, G. B. (1982) 'Intervention Techniques in Pediatric Psychology.' In J. M. Tuma (ed) *Handbook for the Practice of Pediatric Psychology.* New York: Wiley.

Johnstone, K. (1981) *Impro: Improvisation and the Theatre.* London: Methuen.

Kelner, L. B. (1993) *The Creative Classroom.* Portsmouth: Heinemann.

Kim, W. J. (1991) 'Separation Reaction of Psychiatrically Hospitalized Children: A Pilot Study.' *Child Psychiatry and Human Development 22*, 1, 53–67.

Kratochwill, T. R. and Morris, R. J. (eds) (1993) *Handbook of Psychotherapy with Children and Adolescents.* Boston, MA: Allyn and Bacon.

Krietemeyer, B. and Heiney, S. (1992) 'Storytelling as a Therapeutic Technique in a Group for School-aged Oncology Patients.' *Children's Health Care 21*, 14–19.

Landy, R. (1983) 'The Use of Distancing in Drama Therapy.' *The Arts in Psychotherapy 10*, 175–185.

Landy, R. (1990) 'The Concept of Role in Drama Therapy.' *The Arts in Psychotherapy 17*, 223–230.

Landy, R. (1996) *Essays in Drama Therapy: The Double Life.* London: Jessica Kingsley Publishers.

Lowenfeld, M. (1967) *Play in Childhood.* New York: Wiley.

Luthi, M. (1984) *The Fairytale as an Art Form and Portrait of a Man.* Bloomington: Indiana University Press.

McCaslin, N. (1985) *Children and Drama.* New York: David McKay.

McCaslin, N. (1990) *Creative Drama in the Classroom.* London: Longman.

McGlathery, J. M. (ed) (1988) *The Brothers Grimm and Folktale.* Chicago: University of Illinois Press.

McGlathery, J. M. (ed) (1993) *Grimm's Fairy Tales: A History of Criticism on a Popular Classic.* Columbia, SC: Camden House.

Magrab, P. R. (ed) (1986) *Psychological Management of Pediatric Problems.* Baltimore, MD: University Park Press.

Mead, G. H. (1934) *Mind, Self and Society.* Chicago, IL: University of Chicago.

Miles, M. B. and Huberman, A. M. (1984) *Qualitative Data Analysis.* London: Sage.

Millar, S. (1968) *The Psychology of Play.* New York: Penguin.

Moustakos, C. E. (1953) *Children in Play Therapy.* New York: McGraw-Hill.

Murphy, K. and Davidshofer, C. (1988) *Psychological Testing.* Englewood Cliffs, NJ: Prentice Hall.

Pass, M. and Bolig, R. (1993) 'A Comparison of Play Behaviors in Two Child Life Program Variations.' *Children's Health Care 22*, 5–17.

Patton, M. Q. (1990) *Qualitative Evaluation and Research Methods*. London: Sage.

Pellegrino, V. P. (1994) 'The Mask as a Means of Supporting Health Professionals Who Work with People with AIDS.' Ann Arbor, MI: Dissertation Services.

Peppard, M. B. (1971) *Paths through the Forest*. New York: Holt, Rinehart and Winston.

Peter, M. (1995) *Making Drama Special*. London: David Fulton.

Petrillo, M. and Sanger, S. (1972) *Emotional Care of Hospitalized Children*. Philadelphia, PA: J. B. Lippincott.

Phillips, A. (1988) *Winnicott*. Cambridge, MA: Harvard University Press.

Rae, W. and Worchil, F. (1989) 'The Psychosocial Impact of Play in Hospitalized Children.' *The Journal of Pediatric Psychology 14*, 617–627.

Robertson, S. (1982) *Rosegarden and Labyrinth*. Dallas, TX: Spring Publications.

Saar, D. (1997) *The Yellow Boat*. Louisiana: Anchorage Press.

Sarbin, T. (1954) 'Role Therapy.' In G. Lindzey (ed) *Handbook of Social Psychology*, vol. 1. Cambridge: Addison-Wesley.

Schaefer, C. (ed) (1976) *The Therapeutic Use of Child's Play*. New York: Jason Aronson.

Scheff, T. J. (1979) *Catharsis in Healing, Ritual and Drama*. Berkeley, CA: University of California Press.

Segal, L. (ed) (1973) *The Juniper Tree and Other Tales from Grimm*. New York: Farrar, Straus and Giroux.

Siks, G. B. (1983) *Drama with Children*. New York: Harper and Row.

Singer, D. and J. (1990) *The House of Make-Believe*. Cambridge, MA: Harvard University Press.

Slater, B. and Thomas, J. (1983) *Psychodiagnostic Evaluation of Children*. New York: Teacher's College Press.

Somers, J. (1994) *Drama in the Curriculum*. London: Cassell.

South, M. (ed) (1987) *Mythical and Fabulous Creatures*. New York: Greenwood Press.

Spinetto, J. J. (1982) 'The Pediatric Psychologist's Role in Catastrophic Illness: Research and Clinical Issues.' In J. Tuma (ed) *Handbook for the Practice of Pediatric Psychology*. New York: Wiley.

Spolin, V. (1963) *Improvisation for the Theatre*. Evanston, IL: Northwestern University Press.

Stanislavski, C. (1936) *An Actor Prepares*. New York: Theatre Arts Books.

Strasberg, L. (1987) *A Dream of Passion*. New York: Plume.

Swartz, L. (1995) *Dramathemes*. Ontario: Pembroke Publishers.

Swortzell, L. (1992) *Cinderella: The World's Favorite Fairy Tale*. Charlottesville, VA: New Plays.

Szajnberg, N. (1993) 'Psychopathology and Relationship Measures in Children with Inflammatory Bowel Disease and Their Parents.' *Child Psychiatry and Human Development 23*, 3, 215–232.

Tuma, J. M. (ed) (1982) *The Handbook for the Practice of Pediatric Psychology*. New York: Wiley.

Turner, V. (1982) *From Ritual to Theatre: The Human Seriousness of Play*. New York: PAJ.

Van Maanen, J. (1983) *Qualitative Methodology*. London: Sage.

Waelti-Walters, J. (1982) *Fairy Tales and the Female Imagination*. Montreal: Eden Press.

Wallander, J. and Varni, J. (1988) 'Children with Chronic Physical Disorders: Maternal Reports of their Psychological Adjustment.' *Journal of Pediatric Psychology 13*, 197–212.

Wallas, L. (1985) *Stories for the Third Ear*. New York: Norton.

Ward, W. (1952) *Stories to Dramatize*. New Orleans: Anchorage Press.

Watson, R. I. (1951) *The Clinical Method in Psychology*. New York: Harper and Brothers.

Winn, L. (1994) *Post Traumatic Stress Disorder and Drama Therapy*. London: Jessica Kingsley Publishers.

Wood, G. (1977) *Fundamentals of Psychological Research*. Boston, MA: Little, Brown.

Yearsley, M. (1924) *The Folklore of Fairy Tales*. London: Watts.

Yin, R. (1984) *Case Study Research*. Beverly Hills, CA: Sage.

Zahourek, R. P. (ed) (1988) *Relaxation and Imagery*. Philadelphia, PA: Saunders.

Zipes, J. (1987) *Victorian Fairy Tales: The Revolt of the Fairies and Elves*. New York: Methuen.

Zipes, J. (1988) *The Brothers Grimm: From Enchanted Forests to the Modern World*. New York: Routledge.

Zipes, J. (1993) *The Trials and Tribulations of Little Red Riding Hood*. New York: Routledge.

Subject Index

Author Index